"I love this book—a harrowing and some̶ ̶ ̶ning account by a brilliant doctor of how she he̶ ̶ ̶ and soul from a debilitating autoimmun̶ ̶ ̶ ̶iven up on her, with a husband and two ̶ ̶ ̶out of the constraints of Western medic̶ ̶ ̶ ̶ue to health, renewal, and her own true self. This ̶ ̶ ̶̶tten, prescriptive book is going to change—and even save—people's lives."

> —**Anne Lamott**, *New York Times* bestselling author of
> *Bird by Bird* and *Almost Everything*

"*Eat, Pray, Love* meets *Anatomy of an Illness* meets a Deepak Chopra workshop in this engaging, exquisitely written doctor-as-patient memoir. Cynthia Li humbly, humorously, and honestly unearths the roots of her debilitating illness, but the gifts don't stop there. With 15 practical, grounded tips for how to heal, this book also serves as an unconventional, whole health prescription, sure to facilitate the healing journey of others. With raw transparency and the kind of courage we need among both doctors and patients, *Brave New Medicine* charts a new terrain, bridging conventional medicine with functional medicine, nutrition, environmental health, intuition, and spirituality—all in a highly entertaining, hard-earned miracle story."

> —**Lissa Rankin, MD**, *New York Times* bestselling author of
> *Mind Over Medicine* and *The Daily Flame*, and founder of the
> Whole Health Medicine Institute

"In Cynthia Li's spellbinding book, we encounter the moving story of a physician struggling with her own autoimmune illness. Li's writing is so intimate—and so exacting—that it cuts like a knife. She raises fundamental questions about the future of medicine, her own future, and about being a doctor and a patient at the same time. The result is a beautiful book that will be read and remembered for years to come."

> —**Siddhartha Mukherjee**, Pulitzer Prize-winning author of
> *The Emperor of All Maladies*

"Each year brings a new stack of 'how-to' health manuals, but Cynthia Li's book is different. It's a moving, personal—and sometimes unsettling—investigation into the deepest questions surrounding chronic illness. What makes us sick? How do we live with the uncertainty of a mysterious condition? How do we define health in an age when conventional medicine focuses almost exclusively on disease management? The answers Li arrives at in her exploration change her as a person, and the way she practices medicine. Her book is full of wisdom for both health care practitioners and those suffering from chronic illness."

> —**Chris Kresser, MS, LAc**, *New York Times* bestselling author
> of *Unconventional Medicine*

"It is a major concession to admit how much Li's book inspired me, given how deeply skeptical I am about alternative medicine. When Li, a physician herself, develops a terrifying syndrome that regular medicine can't even identify, she becomes her own doctor, charting her symptoms, doing experiments, and seeking help from whoever offers it. Emotionally, she rises from a crouch of defeat to the confident stride of an explorer—and you will find yourself rising with her."

> —**Barbara Ehrenreich**, author of *Natural Causes*, and founder of
> the Economic Hardship Reporting Project

"This is a memoir for our time. Cynthia Li is a superbly trained physician of internal medicine whose life comes to a halt by a life-threatening, complex illness the mainstream medical community doesn't know how to treat. Her struggle is replicated thousands of times over by others who face similar mystery diseases. While the path to recovery is rarely simple, Li's journey and scientific explanations offer hope to many who are suffering. She writes with insight, wisdom, and passion. Her honesty will touch you deeply. Don't miss this book."

> —**Michael Lerner**, author of *Choices in Healing*, and president
> and cofounder of Commonweal

"Cynthia Li is an extraordinary physician with a comprehensive understanding of autoimmune disease as a practitioner and a patient. The insights she provides in this new book are essential for any patient suffering from autoimmunity. Her book challenges the current health care system model that is in such serious need of revision. This is a must-read for anyone suffering from an autoimmune disease."

—**Datis Kharrazian, PhD, DC**, award-winning researcher, clinician, and best-selling author of *Why Do I Still Have Thyroid Symptoms? When My Lab Tests Are Normal*

"Cynthia Li shares a deeply personal and inspiring journey, wherein she falls through the cracks of the conventional medical model but then discovers her own lifesaving path through functional and integrative medicine. Her book also includes an excellent resource filled with practical tips for those who want to learn how to take natural steps to recover their own health and vitality."

—**Akil Palanisamy, MD**, integrative medicine physician, and author of *The Paleovedic Diet*

"Beautifully written, heartbreakingly honest, and deeply inspirational. This is the story of a doctor whose personal experience transforms her view of what it means to be sick, and what it means to truly heal. Millions of people living with autoimmune disease (myself included) will see themselves reflected in these pages."

—**Eileen Laird**, host of *Phoenix Helix*, a podcast dedicated to autoimmune health

"Cynthia Li's book had me hanging onto every word. It's honest and raw, beautifully capturing the day-to-day life of someone living with an invisible illness. But more than that, this book is a conversion story of a doctor breaking into a new way of thinking and living, taking us through well-researched science into time-tested healing principles to show us how to do the same."

—**Dana Trentini, MA, EdM**, founder of the award-winning blog, *Hypothyroid Mom*

"Cynthia Li has written an insightful, captivating account of her own spiral into the depths of a chronic disease, from which prospects of recovery seemed bleak. Li questions the foundational principles learned in her extensive medical training, including the meaning of the term 'health.' Emerging from those dark days, Li has a message of hope for others with similar conditions: autoimmunity can be reversible. There is much to be learned by both patients and health care professionals from this deeply personal account."

—**Ted Schettler, MD, MPH**, science director of the Health
and Environment Science Network, and author of *The Ecology
of Breast Cancer*

"*Brave New Medicine* is a medical memoir as harrowing as it is hopeful. As Cynthia Li battles her own self-doubt and entrenched medical thinking to combat her mysterious illness, she questions everything she thought she knew—from her Western medical training to her traditional Chinese upbringing. Throughout her journey, Li creates the stepping-stones for a new path to health—and emerges with a brave new paradigm for medicine, for her patients, and for herself."

—**Lauren Schiller**, creator and host of *Inflection Point*, a podcast
and public radio show about women, societal change, and the
quest for equality

"In *Brave New Medicine*, Cynthia Li masterfully describes her hard-won transformation from disease to wellness, as she discovers the freedom beyond dogma and formulas, and the wisdom of living the full human experience. She reveals the secret of *healing*, which is very different than *treating*."

—**Master Mingtong Gu**, international teacher, and founder of
The Chi Center

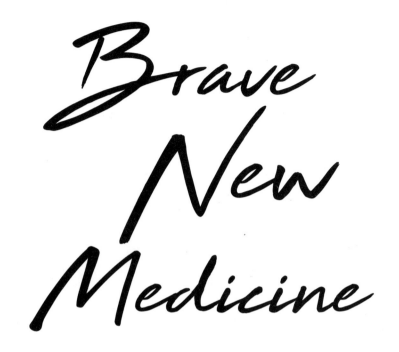

Brave New Medicine

A DOCTOR'S
UNCONVENTIONAL PATH
TO HEALING HER
AUTOIMMUNE ILLNESS

WITHDRAWN

CYNTHIA LI, MD

REVEAL PRESS

AN IMPRINT OF NEW HARBINGER PUBLICATIONS

Publisher's Note

This publication is designed to provide accurate and authoritative information in regard to the subject matter covered. It is sold with the understanding that the publisher is not engaged in rendering psychological, financial, legal, or other professional services. The medical information in this book is provided as an educational resource only, and is not intended to be used or relied upon for any diagnostic or treatment purposes. If expert assistance or counseling is needed, the services of a competent professional should be sought.

The events described in this book are based on the author's memory of real-world situations, as well as oral histories, journals, and personal videos. In some instances, the chronology of events has been changed. To protect privacy, the names and identifying characteristics of the patients and some of the doctors have been changed. Any resemblance to persons living or dead is unintentional and entirely coincidental.

Distributed in Canada by Raincoast Books

Copyright © 2019 by Cynthia Li
Reveal Press
An Imprint of New Harbinger Publications, Inc.
5674 Shattuck Avenue
Oakland, CA 94609
www.newharbinger.com

Cover design by Amy Shoup; Acquired by Catharine Meyers; Edited by Teja Watson; Text design by Michele Waters and Tracy Carlson

Printed in the United States of America

Library of Congress Cataloging-in-Publication Data on file

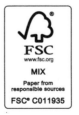 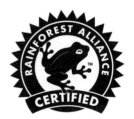

Printed in the United States of America

21   20   19

10   9   8   7   6   5   4   3   2   1   First Printing

For David, Rosa, and Sonia

and

For my parents

Contents

Foreword

In this extraordinary book, Cynthia Li invites us on an odyssey shared by millions: an active life interrupted by a baffling illness. Vibrantly healthy, she was a devoted doctor to underserved patients, a wife, and a mother, living her life to the fullest. But then a physical collapse left her sleepless, dizzy, and housebound for years, even as test after test showed everything as "normal." Halted in midlife by illness, with fear, rage, and despondency threatening her very will to live, Cynthia surrendered her classical training as an internist, and set about rebuilding her medical knowledge from the bottom up.

She illuminates for the reader how doctors are classically trained to think—and why this needs to change. She was taught that health and disease are black-and-white states of being: on one side of a line you're well, and on the other, you're sick. Learning instead that chronic disease is a deeply dynamic and layered process, she stops ignoring her symptoms and, instead, begins a conversation with them. Instead of taking drugs to silence her body, when her heart flutters, she asks, What is it trying to say? Hypersensitivity to light and sounds—What is *that* saying? This intimate conversation with her body sparks the discoveries that lie at the heart of this book.

While we work in different fields—I'm a sociologist and she's a medical doctor—I recognize a common thread in how we work. In the course of researching my last book, on the bitter political divide in our nation, I ventured from my home in liberal Berkeley, California, to deeply conservative towns in the Deep South, to climb an empathy wall dividing people like me from people like them. Cynthia ventures to another unfamiliar territory—the No Man's Land where conventional medicine doesn't go. She creates a bridge between mainstream medicine, time-tested "alternative" practices (many ancient, and in the end, foundational), and cutting-edge science, aiming to personalize medicine even as she broadens it. In a sense, we both start by listening to untold stories, revealing their paradoxes, then looking for answers.

I've witnessed this journey firsthand: the author, I'm honored to say, is my daughter-in-law. Poetically written and bracingly honest, this book highlights new answers—ones that were invisible to me even up close to this agonizing process—and also raises new questions. Why are more and more patients branded as "difficult" even as more and more doctors feel burned out? Are we more estranged from an understanding of health than we realize? Does illness extend beyond the individual to a larger social context, and across generations? What *really* causes disease? And how do we heal? It is through Cynthia's capacity for deep, empathic listening that she reimagines the science and art of healing and gives us a brave new medicine.

—Arlie Russell Hochschild

Prologue: The Difficult Patient

2016

On the ground floor of a major medical center, I was in the bathroom, chanting out loud to myself. *Zhonggg...zhonggg...* These sounds were part of my longstanding qigong practice, but at the moment, I was using them to steady my dizziness. The achiness in my chest wasn't too bad today; neither was the soreness in my muscles. *Linggg...linggg...* As my equilibrium steadied, I looked in the mirror, stood a little taller, and practiced a professional smile. Now I just felt nervous. In fifteen minutes, I would be the guest speaker at Grand Rounds, a conference for doctors across all specialties. The subject of my talk: a new paradigm of medicine.

The auditorium was an icebox, and the chill compounded my nervousness. The lights were dimmed, and doctors lined the lunch buffet in the back. Someone offered me a plate of lasagna, but I declined. Instead, I took a few bites of a honey nut bar and walked toward the podium. The organizer greeted me, and a tech hooked me up with a headset. I rubbed my hands to warm myself. As the doctors seated themselves, I scanned the room. A wall of eyes glared at me like animals in the wild, ready to pounce if I made any false moves—if any of my points were too "alternative."

Then I came across a pair of familiar sea-blue eyes in the front row. My husband, David, had come for moral support. I smiled, took a deep breath, and gave my opening remarks.

"Years ago, I practiced at a hospital like this one. Now, I practice in a very different way. How did I get from there to here? As with most changes in medicine, it began with a patient."

I clicked on the first slide.

"The patient was a thirty-four-year-old female, three months postpartum, who complained of heart palpitations. 'An innocent flutter,' she called it. But the innocence faded when she developed insomnia and rapid weight loss. Her moods became labile, and she grew intolerant of heat. Past medical history—unremarkable. Family history—unremarkable. Social history—no tobacco, alcohol, or drugs." The next slide summarized the patient's labs and imaging studies. "This was a textbook case of postpartum thyroiditis."

The eyes in the audience continued to track me.

"The story didn't end there," I said. "The patient went through a typical course of thyroiditis, but returned a year later, complaining of persistent symptoms. I checked her thyroid numbers, which were normal. I ran some additional labs, which were also normal. She complained that her symptoms were so erratic they frightened her, and at some point, the exhaustion and dizziness kept her housebound. I ran some more tests, which were normal—so I reassured her that she was fine. Numbers don't lie."

My next slide had but one question:

If the tests are normal, does a disease exist?

With that as my backdrop, I stepped away from the podium. "I'd like to see a show of hands. Who here might have run some more tests?"

No response.

"Who might think she was depressed?"

Some rumblings of recognition.

"I screened her for depression, but her test was unremarkable. At this point, who here might refer her to a psychiatrist anyway?"

I nodded and raised my hand. Some hands in the audience went up, too.

"She continued to challenge what I believed to be true, even though it was based on expert guidelines and years of clinical experience. So who here thinks it should have been time to pass her on to another doctor?"

The rumblings increased. I felt like I was standing at a pulpit, my congregation responding with amens.

"There was just one problem."

The room quieted.

"This patient was me."

More than a decade has passed, and I can still feel the ominous flutter. It feels even clearer now than the day it started, because at the time, I had no idea what it meant. The quality was deceptively gentle, like a baby chick ruffling its feathers beneath my breastbone. But in the coming years, this ruffle would escalate into a storm of unimaginable symptoms—dizziness, exhaustion, and profound weakness—making me my own most difficult patient. This difficult patient would break me down, then break me open to new ways of understanding health and disease. She would reveal to me just how layered and dynamic the human body was.

The journey toward optimal health isn't a simple one. It's a mystery embedded in the personal ecosystem of mind, body, and spirit.

Part One

ONE

As a little girl, I never dreamed of becoming a doctor. I'm not sure I dreamed of becoming anything at all, unless princesses and fairies count. I was an "orchid child," a term used in psychology to describe a child who is emotionally and socially sensitive to her environment, in contrast to a "dandelion child," who readily adapts wherever she lands. This meant I would be plugging my nose against foul odors before others even got a whiff. Noises that were average or subtle for others might startle me, including the volume at which people spoke. Sometimes I felt I could even hear their thoughts, and the chatter of their minds was too much.

I preferred to be in quieter spaces, with my Fisher-Price "Little People," and have real people somewhere in the background. Inside a closet or outside under a tree, I would spend entire Saturdays alone creating different scenes, mixing and matching Little People with my crayon drawings, usually of magical kingdoms. The drawings weren't all that special—my princesses wore standard shiny crowns and pink, fluffy dresses—but in my imagination, they came alive. Their wands helped find lost puppies, and the hearts on their capes made sad children smile.

Around the time I was six, I woke from my imaginary world to the real one. Here, living things got hurt, and they wouldn't just get better with magic. My two younger brothers were chasing each other down the hall one day, and the younger one ran into a door and slit his pinky toe, making a bloody mess all over the beige carpet. My brothers were screaming, my mother and older sister were frantic, and I ran back into my room, paralyzed by the noise and tension. Another time, the black stray cat that lived near our house came meowing up our driveway. Her cry sounded frailer than usual, so I gave her what I was eating, a Milk

Dud. She chomped it down, but started to choke and gag and writhe until, finally, the chocolate-caramel goo dislodged from her throat.

And then there were the roly-polies. One day when I was hanging out under the cedar tree, I spotted a pill bug whose shell was crushed. Wanting to create a sanctuary for "Roly," I grabbed an empty pickle jar from the house. In went twigs, soil, and a few leaves for a bed. Roly looked lonely, so I collected several other pill bugs, dropped them in, then closed the lid tight, lest anything try to harm them. Three days passed. Or perhaps it was a week. *The roly-polies!* I raced to say hello to them, picking a handful of leaves along the way. The jar released a stench. The bugs were curled up and unmoving.

"How come they won't wake up?" I asked my parents. They peeked inside. "Oh, they're dead." *Dead?* The sound of that word scared me. The hard *d* at the start, followed by *ehhh*, the sound of struggle, then a second *d* bringing it to a hard close.

Whether it really happened or it's only how I remember it now, the colors of my childhood began to fade—as though someone had taken a big eraser to the rich hues and textures and left only the hard black outlines. My emotions seem to have lost their texture, too, because while I can remember minute details of events that happened, I can't seem to recall much about how I felt.

I have tried to resurrect those emotions by studying photographs of myself. They show a young Chinese girl with a looped pigtail atop her head, the expression on her downward-tilting face enigmatic in some, wooden in others. What I recall most is laughter—not coming from me, but directed at me. This was often followed by someone saying, "Don't be so sensitive." It didn't matter who was saying it; I knew they were right. My sensitivities hindered me. Desperate to learn another way, I began to fill in these hard, black outlines—not with emotion, but with information. Anything to help me survive.

I came from a family of survivors. My mother and father were born in China, during a time of chaos and upheaval. China was at war with Japan, forcing their families to flee to Taiwan. They endured extraordinary hardships, many of which remain unspoken to this day. My father's family left everything behind, including his baby sister—entrusted to neighbors, for fear the journey by train and boat was too dangerous. In Taiwan, his father served as a military judge. While this brought honor to their family, they remained poor. Their house had dirt floors and they bred chickens to sell. Their diet consisted mostly of white rice; chicken, their primary meat, was eaten once a month at most. My father's mother worked in a cigarette factory, and his older brother peddled cigarettes after school.

When I struggled to understand how they overcame all their challenges, my grandfather would usually say something like *Huo dao lao, xue dao lao* (Live long, learn long). A good education had been my father's ticket to a better life—he studied hard, got into Taiwan University, Taiwan's preeminent university, and after a year of compulsory military training, made his way to graduate school in America.

My mother's family settled in Taiwan with more ease. Her father was a high-ranking railroad commissioner and her mother—my Puo Puo—was a doctor. It was rare for a woman to be educated in those days, rarer yet for her to study medicine. And even rarer to study Western medicine. Beyond her field, obstetrics and gynecology, I didn't know much about her work life, nor did I think to ask. I was more interested in how my Puo Puo, at five feet tall and eighty-five pounds, with a soft glamour reminiscent of classic movie stars, could have such harsh rules for her children: no listening to the radio, no playing with friends after school, no reading of books or magazines or newspapers except those assigned in class.

I asked my mother how she felt about all this when I was in middle school. "Children are to obey their parents," she said, "so I obeyed." Chinese people didn't talk about feelings, because it risked burdening others, so I didn't press on. What mattered, my mother said, was that her obedience paid off. She made her way to Taiwan University, which was where she met my father.

When I was born, my parents were new immigrants to America. Their marriage was a traditional one. My father had completed a PhD in electrical engineering and took a job with IBM in upstate New York, working long days to support the six of us and send money to his parents. My mother managed the home: shopping, cooking, cleaning, and childcare. It wasn't until I became a mother myself that I understood how exhausted she must have been, with four children sandwiched between five years.

By Chinese custom, they called my sister The Eldest. My brothers were Number Three and The Youngest. I was Number Two. Following The Eldest by fifteen months, I mostly looked to her on how to act. Since we looked alike and had the same voice, people often mistook us for twins. But year after year, my sister was the favorite of all her teachers, while year after year, I disappointed the same teachers. In the evenings, I would be reading the comics, while my sister watched and discussed the evening news with our father. When Connie Chung became an anchorwoman, my sister set her ambitions on journalism. My sister's mind had a spark, her spirit a boldness. Next to her, I felt small, unseen. I was Number Two in a world that favored Number Ones.

Still, I knew my parents loved me. Not because they kissed or hugged me or said "I love you," but because they prayed for me. My parents met at Taiwan University, during a Christian retreat. God was the foundation of their love, and the foundation of our family. They emphasized God above politics, money, and even education. When we moved to Austin, Texas, my parents founded a Chinese evangelical church, the first of its kind in the area. My father was a deacon, and my mother a Sunday school teacher. We attended church every Sunday without fail. For the annual Christmas pageants, we dressed in complementary outfits, singing hymns in Mandarin and English. On family trips, my parents found services for us to attend—and this was before GPS, cell phones, and Yelp, so they had to put in some serious effort to find them. Once, at the Grand Tetons, my father woke us up at the crack of dawn and we drove for over an hour along mountain roads to a tiny, stand-alone chapel. I searched this tiny chapel for proof of God, as I searched all the churches we visited. But even high in the mountains, God, who was supposedly Love, eluded me. Love as a whole often felt that way to me—an invisible cloud in the sky.

In Sunday school, we watched A Thief in the Night, a film in which a woman ran through the streets, looking for her family, who had vanished with millions of others in the rapture, while she, a nonbeliever, was left behind. By the end, my legs, fingers, and insides would be quivering with fear. Other weeks, my teachers would remind us that Mormons and Catholics and Buddhists were cultists and therefore destined for hell—not to mention the unmarried couples who confessed their sexual acts to the congregation. I became terrified that my beliefs weren't enough, that I wasn't enough, and come the real rapture I would be left behind. Figuring my fears had something to do with my sensitivities—a defect—I armored myself with Bible verses.

Then there was school. I grew up in the outskirts of Austin in the late-1970s, my siblings and I among some of the only non-white children in our elementary school. The kids who played with me were the left-behind bunch. When teams were picked, I was usually picked last, along with a girl with mild cerebral palsy, and a boy who was severely overweight. I was often teased for my eyelids being "Mongoloid."

When I turned ten, an opportunity arose to change all this. My mother gave my sister and me permission to walk home from school. There were responsibilities that came with this privilege: "Come straight home, don't talk to strangers, and stick with Jennifer." Jennifer was a popular girl in my grade who lived across the street and already knew the route. This was my chance to hang out with someone I admired.

One afternoon, halfway home, we noticed a vacant lot. Jennifer suggested we check it out. My sister wasn't interested, and continued on. I wavered between pleasing my mother and pleasing Jennifer. My sister was already a block ahead when I hollered that I would see her at home. Beyond the tall grasses and shrubs was a glorious patch of blackberries. Jennifer glanced at me, wide-eyed and wide-mouthed. A magical kingdom! We picked, we ate, and we picked some more, tangled in the brambles. I was untucking my shirt to use as a pouch to bring some berries home for my mother, when I remembered: my mother! Ten minutes had ballooned into two hours.

She was waiting on the front steps when I arrived, my mouth stained dark purple, hands scratched from thorns, T-shirt dirty. She had been sick with worry, having called Jennifer's mother, other neighbors, and almost the police. My mother gave my sister and me a good paddling: me, for obvious reasons, my sister, for leaving me behind. *Gai si*, my mother cursed; translated directly, this meant "You should die" (though many years later I would learn it wasn't literal, more like a firm "damn it"). Primed by evangelical visions of hell and a God too high to reach, hearing Jennifer snicker behind the screen door, then having my sister dig her fingernails into my skin for getting her in trouble, and having nowhere to turn because I knew my parents went through much greater hardships than I ever did, I thought I *should* die. I sure wanted to.

No matter how I tried, I continued to miss the mark. The threat of backsliding haunted me, so I began to pray day and night, in atonement for my imperfections. This sense of helplessness continued until, one day in the sixth grade, something in the newspaper caught my attention. It was a photo of Arnold Schwarzenegger as the Terminator, wearing sunglasses and flexing his biceps, with the following caption:

What doesn't kill you makes you stronger.

I cut out the photo and taped it into my diary, vowing to be more like that. I was older now. I was done with feeling weak.

My first strategy was to use my Terminator mantra to develop a thicker skin. My grandfather had used sayings to guide his life, and my parents had used Bible verses. I recited mine every morning before school. My second strategy was to control my sensitivities. I trained my mind to focus on what was useful. I finished all my chores (often my siblings', too), practiced piano and violin, and did all my homework. I followed rules, and asked my father to teach me some habits he had learned in the military. "Early to rise, early to bed," he said. And if I made my bed, that would start my day off right. It wasn't a miracle cure, but by getting my surroundings in order, my life seemed to have more order, too.

Then I went through a growth spurt. From the time we were little, the elders in our church would openly comment on our physical features—as the Chinese do, with amazing directness for a culture otherwise steeped in indirectness—like my sister and I having lucky nose bridges and cheekbones. But when I shot up to five-foot-seven, they remarked, "If you get any taller, no man will marry you." I did grow taller, to five-foot-nine, a head above my mother and a half-head above my sister. I slouched to make myself appear smaller.

I kept returning to my singular question: How could I build a thicker skin? Since I wasn't the star student my sister was, I developed my extracurricular activities, adding French horn to the piano and violin, and taking Latin as well as Spanish. I tried out for basketball, but lacked the coordination; instead, I joined the track team. I kept myself busy enough that I wouldn't think about my sensitivities. Despite my efforts, a semester shy of high school graduation, I still found myself lost. I had no desire to do anything with my life. No curiosity or creativity. And unbeknownst to my parents, no plans to go to college.

Then one day in the spring, I received a postcard in the mail from the University of Texas—the local university, twenty miles from our house. They were launching a new incentive for enrollment. For those who graduated in the top ten percent of their class, the application was as simple as checking boxes on the very postcard I held in my hand. A check here, a check there, and I was enrolled. I can't recall if I felt happy or excited. I think I was simply relieved to have some direction in my life.

And as it turned out, college opened up a whole new world. The campus was teeming with fifty thousand students of every race, color, and culture, and for the first time in my life, I felt I belonged somewhere. I lived in an apartment with a friend from high school, and made new friends easily. Two months in, a fellow freshman named Charles asked me to study with him. He was smart, handsome—and tall. We soon fell in love. Filled with wonder, I rode around campus on the back of his (my boyfriend's!) motorcycle, my arms around his waist, a changed person.

With newfound love and independence, the trees looked greener, the sky looked bluer. And my classes were more enjoyable. In fact, I found I loved learning. I read constantly: Homer, Rilke, Kierkegaard, all the classics. I discovered that Nietzsche was the mastermind behind the

Terminator philosophy, and laughed at the mistakes of my younger self. I read Jung for sheer pleasure, and recognized in him my existential wrestling about God. By sophomore year, I stopped going to church. I couldn't understand how the Bible intersected with real life. To my parents' horror, I declared myself agnostic.

My devotion was to knowledge. I became a purist: for example, taking four semesters of Russian because I felt the works of Tolstoy should be read in their original language. My memorization skills came in handy for verb conjugations and noun declensions. This moved me toward becoming a linguist or language teacher. Then, for my junior year science credit, I chose Organic Chemistry, not knowing that this was the notorious weed-out class for pre-med students, most of whom had set their ambitions on medicine at the same age I was playing with Little People. Since I didn't have the academic pressure, the subject matter illuminated how chemicals formed intricate bonds and obeyed give-and-take laws of science, speaking a romantic language of their own. I excelled. At the end of the semester, my study partner said, "Have you ever thought about medical school?"

The idea had never crossed my mind. But now, night after night, I explored this question, my mind volleying between yes and no. Yes— think of all the people I could help. No—I lacked the ambition. Yes— think of the surprise my parents would have if I, Number Two, fulfilled the Chinese parent's dream.

Excited, I called them. "What do you think about medical school?"

"For who?"

"Me!" I imagined confetti falling from the sky.

Instead, silence. When they finally spoke, it was a restrained "wonderful." Interpreting their lukewarm reaction as my parents doubting that I was strong or smart enough, I didn't discuss it further with them.

I asked Charles what he thought.

"My brother's in medical school," he said, "and it's grueling. I don't think women should really work outside the—"

"Please don't finish that sentence."

Two months later, I broke up with Charles.

The question continued to press on me. *Could* I do it if I chose to? I made special arrangements to get my answer. On a Saturday before dawn, I had my cup of coffee, drove to the morgue, and entered through the back door. There, on the table, was the corpse of a young Latina woman who had died a few hours earlier, the cause unknown but a drug overdose suspected. Her body was so fresh that she looked like she was merely dozing. Jet-black hair, olive skin, clumpy mascara, hot pink nail polish. The pathologist investigated her body, organ by glistening organ. Brain, unremarkable. Heart, unremarkable. On through the liver, the spleen, the intestines, until every organ had been examined and weighed, the details recorded.

If I had any visceral reactions, I managed to suppress them, and was proud of my thick skin. After the pathologist reassembled her organs and covered her body with a white sheet, I half expected the woman to step off the table and get on with her life.

For the rest of the weekend, I couldn't shake the image of the dead woman. What had her pain been? And could this tragedy have been prevented? On Sunday evening, my roommate and I attended a party on campus. With a beer in hand and Duran Duran blasting in the background, I sunk into an ottoman in the corner. In everyone I observed, I only saw the dead woman. When a large housefly buzzed around, I saw her miniaturized face on it, too. In a stream of tipsy consciousness, the housefly evoked the roly-polies of a different time, which evoked the choking cat, my brother's bleeding toe, and on and on. Hell wasn't in the afterlife. It was here, now.

To become a doctor wasn't a choice for me. It was a calling.

TWO

My classes at UT Southwestern Medical School in Dallas started in full force, with three times the density and pace of my undergraduate classes. Lectures and labs began daily at eight a.m. Our professors included Nobel Prize–winning researchers, and doctors named Great Teachers by the National Institutes of Health. I was blown away by this noble lineage. Somehow, I had become a part of it.

From the outset, the scientific method was the gold standard. *Ask a question. Gather background data. Construct a hypothesis. Conduct an experiment. Analyze the data. Draw conclusions.* Then repeat as necessary, with a better design. In clinical care, the best study design was the randomized, controlled trial, or RCT, where participants were randomly divided into groups to compare different drugs or interventions. The RCT systematized large, diverse groups of people. And it controlled for life's variables.

By the first semester's end, my focus had already shifted. The suffering of people everywhere would have to wait. For now, I had to live up to the demand of academic excellence. I recorded a covenant from the Hippocratic oath into my journal and vowed to guard it with my entire being:

> I will respect the hard-won scientific gains
> of those physicians in whose steps I walk.

My class had two hundred students in total, about half men and half women. Within days, I recognized some kindred spirits. One was Kurt. He was a striking young man from West Texas who, during our first conversation, had joked, "I'm a recovering Catholic." I laughed, reassured that this stranger shared a common experience with me.

During test weeks, our classmates would be busy cramming their heads full of pathology and biochemistry factoids. Kurt and I were, too, but we took regular study breaks at Chili's or Pizza Hut to explore the larger human condition. He might bring along Ayn Rand's *Atlas Shrugged* or Shakespeare, and I, Homer's *The Odyssey*. Sometimes we looked through *The Far Side* comics for laughs. There wasn't any pretentiousness about it; we always had more questions than answers. And we felt we could always fall back on the scientific method if things got too messy. That is, do our best to control life's variables. Before long, we were deeply in love.

In school, I was eager to apply the scientific method to patient care, but first I had to learn the basics of the History and Physical. "A good H&P," my professor declared, "will tell you 90 percent of what you need to know." This was Dr. Seymour Eisenberg, a professor emeritus who had trained in the era before high-tech diagnostics, electronic health records, and complex insurance schemes. His H&Ps were an art form. He had, in fact, taught his system to the current chairman of the internal medicine department, among other distinguished faculty. Though he beamed warmth and compassion, I feared him, out of the utmost respect.

When I took a special elective to sharpen my H&P skills, Dr. Eisenberg would receive my reports and lift them up and down on his palm, as if to weigh them. He had high expectations, and if the reports were too thin, he would return them with a smile that said *You can do better.* Once accepted, my H&Ps would be marked up like an English paper: the punctuation corrected, the sentences completed, and the modifiers put in the right places. By the end, my history-taking was near perfection.

To learn the P of the H&P, we started in anatomy lab. The cadavers, preserved in formaldehyde, looked more like wax dummies than deceased humans. During late-night dissections, my team would eat dinner there, using hemostats to find the cranial nerves, all twelve of them, memorizing their names, functions, and location. I often felt lightheaded, sometimes dizzy. It was the strong fumes, I presumed— they were so strong, one of my lab-mates required a heavy-duty respirator for her asthma. Why was I having vertigo, though? I would brush it aside, reminding myself, *What doesn't kill you makes you stronger.*

To put together the whole H&P, we went through a Clinical Skills Evaluations course. First, a dynamic team of psychologists and doctors demonstrated a proper patient interview and physical exam. We followed along with handouts, written out like a play script. Later, we took our skills to the Patient Lab, where we practiced comprehensive H&Ps on actors who had memorized a script for a particular ailment, including a full pelvic exam on women whose mock intake suggested gynecologic issues. My face turned crimson in front of my assigned group. But in the end, the actor-patient and I emerged more or less unscathed.

These types of dress rehearsals prepped us for our hospital rotations, four-week sessions through the different specialties. I started with trauma surgery. When the first morning started off slow, I tried suturing. A needle driver in one hand and a headlamp on my forehead, I made continuous stitches with a shiny blue thread. Then my pager went off. Startled, I lost control of the needle and stabbed the skin. My patient didn't complain, though—I was suturing a navel orange. I left it wounded and unsewn in the student lounge, rushing toward the elevators.

I grew nervous, not knowing what awaited me in the emergency room. To keep calm, I rattled off recent mnemonics I had learned—like the five Ws for the causes of post-operative fever: Wind, Water, Wound, Walking, and Wonder drug—until the cacophony of sounds in the ER silenced me. Sirens blared. Gurneys flew. Voices yelled. Stunned, I found my team—a senior surgery resident, a junior resident, an intern, and three medical students—and a triage nurse informed us, "A high-speed MVA."

"A high-speed what?" That wasn't covered in the mnemonics I knew.

"Motor vehicle accident," my resident said, slapping into my hands a long, thin tube wrapped in a sterile plastic bag. "Slide it into her nose and push it down her throat." He pointed to a patient on a gurney and made an arc with his hands.

This was a nasogastric tube. Placed correctly, it would pass through the nose down to the stomach, thereby protecting a semiconscious or unconscious patient from inhaling stomach contents in case they vomited. Eager to be useful, I lubed the N-G tube, and attempted to insert it into the patient's right nostril. I pushed upward, but she swatted me and knocked it out.

I tried not to get worked up. I was treating a person this time, not a navel orange. But I also saw that her injury wasn't serious. So I set aside the tube.

My junior resident entered, his brow scrunched. "Why isn't the tube in?"

"She refused it."

"Who's in charge here?" he barked.

I hesitated for a second, then thought, *He's right, I'm in charge.* I ordered two nursing aides to restrain the patient and tried again. She flailed and whimpered as I struggled with the tube. Drops of blood surrounded her nose, and saliva streaked her hair. A wave of nausea gripped me, but before I heaved, I managed to control it. With a little more force, the tube moved past the point of resistance. Done! I secured it to her cheek with tape and asserted, "It's for your own good."

When the emergency room settled down, my senior resident called our team into a huddle. He reviewed the events of the morning.

"Why was the N-G tube necessary for my patient?" I asked.

"It wasn't," my resident said. "But this is how you learn—see one, do one, teach one. Now you're ready to teach someone else. Got it?"

No, I didn't get it. But I was eager to be a good student, and felt too inexperienced to question my superiors. So I just nodded.

He taught us more lists and mnemonics, and I jotted them all down. They were useful for passing tests, but even more for clarity of thought during moments of crisis. With the several additional traumas that came through the ER overnight, my residents handled each case without a hitch. They taught me to suture an actual laceration, and let me assist in complex procedures like central lines and chest tubes. I studied how they moved, spoke, and executed. I wanted to know how they did it without the constant queasiness I felt.

Dawn came, signaling the end of our shift. My team had breakfast at the McDonald's in the hospital lobby. I pulled the senior resident aside.

"How long did it take you to get used to this?"

"Get used to what?" he said, munching on his McMuffin.

There was no inner process for this line of work. What mattered was how we performed. Don't overthink; act swiftly, and do as you're told, or as the rules demand. This was the same strategy my parents had used to succeed. And here, we were talking about saving lives. No room for ambivalence or sentimentality.

After surgery, the other core rotations followed—internal medicine, pediatrics, obstetrics-gynecology, family medicine, and psychiatry. The hours were long, the learning curve steep, but the camaraderie was unmatched. Post-shift, exhausted teammates would look after each other, pitching in to complete the remaining workload. Usually, the post-call team would doze during lunchtime conferences, their heads bobbing as if in hearty agreement with each talking point. "Why don't you sleep a little?" a classmate would say, giving me permission to doze. But my mind would usually be awake. Wired. My calf muscles would also be sore, like I had just run a marathon. Being in my late twenties, I thought these symptoms were mere annoyances and tried to ignore them. No room for softness here, either.

Before graduation, Kurt and I got engaged. We stayed in Dallas for our residencies: pediatrics for him, internal medicine for me. Internal medicine was the specialty of chronic conditions. Congestive heart failure, gastrointestinal bleeds, hepatitis, pneumonia, diabetes—anything that could be treated without surgery. Each specialty had its distinct "personality," and what drew me to internal medicine was the way internists thought. They observed the body as a puzzle to be solved, and were therefore premiere diagnosticians.

Internists would use a detailed H&P, pertinent test results, and clinical experience to arrive at a diagnosis. If the number of possible diagnoses was overwhelming, I would remember what Dr. Eisenberg had taught me: "Common things are common, uncommon things are uncommon." Focus on the more likely ones, then do tests to rule out disorders, one by one. The process could be tedious, but the diagnosis was paramount. Without one, there was no treatment plan.

On morning rounds, I would present to the attending faculty the cases we had admitted the previous night. The faculty would pepper the medical students with questions on the pathological mechanisms for x or y disease. This was a good refresher for me, too, because once we made the transition from lecture hall to hospital, most of our focus was on drugs and procedures. Different lists to be memorized—first-line drugs, second-line, and third-; the criteria for clot-busting drugs; the criteria for emergency cardiac catheterization; and so on. There seemed to be a pill for every ill. During my second and third years of residency, I served as the medicine "pit boss," working alongside the surgery pit boss to run the entire ER. My white coat was fraying at the edges, the pockets were sagging, and it was no longer white. But these were my badges of courage. I felt invincible in medicine, in life, and in myself.

Until the unthinkable happened.

It was a little after midnight on a clear winter night. Kurt was driving from a late dinner to a friend's house when he lost control of his car, skidding head-on into an oak tree in the middle of the road. And just like that, he was dead. Like the Latina woman at the autopsy. Like the dozens of patients I had pronounced dead in the hospital. I had been working an overnight shift at the veterans hospital, and my roommate broke the news to me the next morning. The grief felt like lye in my throat, first burning, then choking. All I remember from those initial days was an endless cycle of crying and dry heaving, feeling betrayed by Kurt driving too fast and after drinking, and yearning to be with the friends who were with him that night, the last ones to see him alive.

Three hundred medical students, residents, and faculty gathered for his funeral at St. Rita's Catholic Church. The collective grief, especially that reflected in his parents' eyes, was too much for me to bear. I wanted to run to my room like I had as a child, but I had to sit there. Listening to the dean of student affairs give the eulogy, then a cousin, and friends. To get through that eternity, I scanned the church from windows to altar to vaulted ceiling to empty doorways, searching and searching for Kurt.

The day after, I went with Kurt's family to sort through his belongings. After all the time I had considered myself agnostic, I now found myself consumed by the questions of souls, wondering whether the hard *d*'s in *dead* were as final as they sounded. Huddled by his closet, the scent of his sweat still in his clothes, I asked his parents what they believed.

"Souls live on after the body dies," his mother said. Her face was puffy, her eyes moist. "Kurt's been playing jokes on us, like drawing the curtains in our living room. It's just like him to do that from the other side, isn't it?" She gave a forced chuckle. I looked to his father. He was a cardiologist. A scientist. A rational thinker. But he didn't contradict her.

As we sorted through Kurt's medical books, I recalled a patient from a year earlier: green eyes, sunken cheeks, fragile skin upon fragile bones. She had metastatic lung cancer, and we had admitted her for pneumonia and pain control. I had never before encountered anyone so close to the edge, and it frightened me. At the end of my exam, she said in a wisp of breath, "I'm not afraid of death." I sat down and listened. She spoke of the movie *Braveheart*, a Scottish legend of love and loss. "I've never felt such freedom as I do now."

"How?" I had wondered, astonished at her sense of peace.

"Because I can see my sister and mother waiting for me in the light." I hadn't known what to make of it then, and I didn't know now. There was something comforting about the notion of souls living on. But souls that moved about the living room, playing pranks?

I wanted to believe. And I didn't want to believe.

By dusk, we finished sorting the important things. The only items I kept were some letters, photos, and an assortment of Kurt's ID cards and ticket stubs. I placed everything in a shoebox, feeling like I had just shoved Kurt's enormous spirit into a tiny, cardboard compartment. Once in a while, I would remove the lid to give it (him) some breathing space. As for the engagement ring, I threaded it onto a chain and wore it around my neck, low-down, hidden close to my heart.

After a couple of weeks, I resumed my ninety-hour work weeks. When I got hit with a horrible case of mono, I continued to work through it. I was twenty-eight. This was the only way I knew to keep the grief from eating me alive. The familiar rhythms of patient care, the ethos of pragmatism and rationality, and the ability to resuscitate patients—to postpone death itself—gave me a sense of empowerment. I completed my residency with distinction. Restless to leave Texas, I opened a map of the United States and scanned it for places far away in both geography and culture. Somewhere to find anonymity. To look forward, not back. To get a fresh start.

THREE

2001

I moved to San Francisco. My first job was at a primary care clinic in a large medical center. Most of my training had been hospital-based, so outpatient medicine was a whole new terrain. I had naively expected a gentle initiation, with ample time to research and consult with my colleagues. But from the moment I received my ID badge, I had more than three thousand patients assigned to my practice. Phone messages demanded timely answers, and a typical day meant fifteen to twenty appointments. I donned my white coat and gave it my best effort. The cases were lower in acuity than in the hospital, which made things easier. The drug protocols were also laid out: which antibiotics for which infections, which inhalers or steroids for which lung condition, which anti-inflammatories and muscle relaxants for which musculoskeletal pains. Gradually, outpatient medicine felt straightforward—on some days, even rote.

On top of this full-time schedule, I took overnight shifts in the hospital twice a month. For twenty-four hours, I would carry the internal medicine pager and assess patients in the ER. Whereas in residency I had a team to consult with—to say nothing of sharing the psychological load—here, I was on my own. Chest pain, rule out heart attack. Diabetic crisis, hydrate and stabilize. Cellulitis, prescribe antibiotics, IV, and oral. Back to back, nonstop, with five more waiting. By the time the sun rose, I would feel wasted. Muscles sore and head dizzy, I still had a half-day's clinic to endure before going home.

Six months in, enough time had passed that my clinic patients were calling or returning for the same complaints. The ibuprofen didn't work for the pain, the antidepressants had too many side effects, or the antihistamine-decongestants didn't help the sinusitis. More relief, they demanded. More options. More answers. Okay, I said, referring them to specialists when appropriate. Inevitably, some would return with no answers. This kind of nowhere-to-go conundrum didn't happen in the hospital because, well, patients could always go *somewhere*—home or a skilled nursing facility. Now, as the primary doctor, I felt I carried my patients' cumulative frustrations, along with all the other demands.

"How do you do it?" I asked a seasoned colleague.

He peered around a tall stack of charts. "You'll get used to it. There are workshops, you know." He was talking about building resilience and preventing burnout, which was a serious problem. One third to half of all doctors reported emotional exhaustion, cynicism, depersonalization, or feelings of decreased effectiveness.

One workshop I attended was called "Managing Difficult Patients." The presenter stepped up, his posture erect, his voice deep. He started with a formal definition of the "difficult patient" as one who (1) didn't comply with doctors' orders, (2) challenged authority with anger, (3) sought drugs, or (4) exaggerated for a secondary gain. "If your patient comes with a list of multiple complaints," he said, "it's important that you set your boundaries up front. Explain that there's only time for one or two issues in a fifteen-minute appointment." For most of the workshop, we role-played patient and doctor scenarios.

In the clinic, though, it was harder. Many of the chief complaints were vague, the possible diagnoses vast, and the screening tests often negative. The complaint I dreaded most was fatigue. Without a clear cause, the default diagnosis was always "stress," and the treatment was stress management: work less, relax more—not what patients wanted to hear. Some patients brought in wild ideas from the Internet. One patient came in saying, "I'm exhausted all the time. I'm also getting these terrible headaches once a month, and they're causing me to miss a few days of work. And I'm having the worst trouble with my hemorrhoids."

"I understand," I said, recalling the techniques from the workshop. "I'd like to address all of your concerns, but try to pick out one or two for today."

Sighing, she agreed to focus on the fatigue.

I went through a checklist of symptoms for common causes of fatigue, namely anemia, diabetes, thyroid disorders, and depression.

Heavy menstrual bleeds? "Not really."

Blood in the stool? "No."

Black stools? "No."

Cold body temperature? "Maybe?"

Constipation? "A little."

Changes in weight? "No."

Increased thirst, hunger, or urination? "No."

Crying spells, loss of interest in pleasure? "No, and no."

Her physical exam was unremarkable. Not knowing what else to do, I pulled out a requisition slip for basic blood tests to rule out various conditions. If abnormal, we would have something to treat. If normal, everything was okay. I glanced at the clock, seeing that I was five minutes late for my next patient. As I stood up, the patient tugged at my coat.

"Dr. Li, I'm wondering if you can request another test."

This caught me by surprise. In the hospital setting, patients didn't request tests—plenty of tests were already being performed, and some patients asked for *fewer* tests. I felt challenged. Wasn't she seeking *my* expertise?

"I'm worried I could have chronic mono," she said.

I paused for a second. Now she was challenging my patience, too. Mono was short for the viral infection mononucleosis, which I had diagnosed many times, and from which patients fully recovered. "Mono is an acute infection. I'm afraid it's not chronic."

She bit her lower lip. "I read online…"

The World Wide Web was a mixed bag of sound science and pseudoscience. I wanted her to feel better, but not at the risk of my integrity. I politely declined her request.

After work, I walked to my car with a colleague.

"Today I had a patient ask me about 'leaky gut,'" he said. "Another one of those quack diagnoses floating around the Web."

"How 'bout 'chronic mono'?"

We shared a laugh. But in my car, I began to feel claustrophobic. The patient complaints were on one side and my limited tools were on the other, closing in. I knew I had done everything right, according to the standard of care. What if her labs were normal, as I anticipated them to be? Then what? I longed for more built-in time to research, examine each patient, and collaborate with my colleagues. Perhaps it was as my senior colleague had said, that I had to get used to how things were in real-world medicine.

On the long commute home, I recalled the way I had been trained: There was a distinct line between health and disease. *Here* you're well, *there* you're not. The line could be a number, a diagnostic test, or a set of criteria. Sometimes the line would move, depending on the latest clinical guidelines. But either way, if you met *x*, then you had *y*; if you didn't, you didn't. And if a patient didn't qualify for a diagnosis, my job was to monitor him until he crossed over from *here* to *there*. Then I would prescribe the appropriate treatment.

Nearing home, I reassured myself that I was doing all I could for my patients. Still, I felt something missing from this paradigm. What exactly, I couldn't put my finger on.

Outside of work, I enjoyed the novelty of San Francisco. I didn't know many people in the area, but a friend from college had an open room in her house in the Inner Sunset district. I moved in, along with Happy, my twelve-year-old Pekingese. The floors creaked, the walls were paper-thin, and the nearest laundromat was three blocks away. But I didn't mind. I preferred experiences over material things. The house was within walking distance of world-class restaurants and Golden Gate Park, and a short streetcar hop to Ocean Beach. Three of us lived together, two doctors and a teacher, all from Texas, all single. Many nights, we would stay up late, sharing the events of the day. On weekends, we would compare notes on our dates. New Year's Eve, we threw a party with a wig theme. Sporting a blonde bob and a beauty mark, I toasted with my roommates, "To my new, cozy family."

Despite the cozy family, Happy, and a few friends at work, I was growing detached from myself and others. My grief from Kurt's death felt like a lead ball in my center, oozing low-grade toxicity. It wasn't enough to put me into a deep depression, but it infused a general grayness over life's textures. Sometimes I would ride the cable cars in Chinatown to study the tourists, mystified at how they could look so happy, trying to detect undercurrents of pain beneath their happy masks. Dating was a nice diversion, but other thirty- and forty-somethings seemed to be looking for "The Relationship." I was far from it, and never wanted to explain my past. My friends from Texas understood me better, but I stopped returning their phone calls. The grayness lifted during my commutes, when I chatted with the empty passenger seat. "Kurt, what d'you think Dante meant when he described the deepest level of hell as frozen?"

Traveling also added splashes of color. Greece. Italy. Cuba. Whenever I returned, though, the grayness was sure to follow.

I searched out local sanctuaries. St. Anne's was a Catholic church I passed on my morning jogs—old, grand, cotton-candy pink, and taking up most of a block. I never thought I would consider a church a true refuge, but one morning, a compulsion seized me as I jogged by, and I pulled on the door handle to find it unlocked. Inside was a glorious palace, also pink, with high ceilings and stained-glass windows along both sides, topped by an intricate dome above the altar. I sat down in the back pew for ten or fifteen minutes, my first time in a Catholic church since Kurt's funeral. I can't say I felt closer to God; I don't know if I was even looking for Him. But I felt closer to Kurt, like he and I were visiting a cathedral in Florence, and after leaving the church, maybe we would find a *gelateria* to sample some *gianduia* or *cioccolato*.

My other sanctuary was the beach. Unlike their southern counterparts, Northern California beaches were often chilly and damp, and seagulls outnumbered the people. Anyone brave enough to swim usually wore a full wetsuit. I was content to stay warm and dry, resting under a woolly throw with my journal or a book. After dusk, I would sit in my car, watching the bonfires: groups of people, young and old, huddled around the flames, warming their hands and roasting hot dogs. If the winds were right, I could catch pieces of their conversations, more often than not an exchange of ideas, like inventing the next tech breakthrough or solving the homelessness crisis. Everyone in this city seemed intent on changing the world.

In late October during election season, a friend invited me to a fund-raiser downtown. A boyishly handsome man was at the microphone, proclaiming the need for greater independence from fossil fuels. His wheat-colored hair was tousled and he wore a T-shirt that said GET SOME SUN, over a pair of blue jeans that fell an inch too short. "The solution is solar!" he raved.

Not being drawn to politics, I was unexpectedly struck. His bold ideas and an absence of slickness pulled me out of my grayness into curiosity. The folks behind me clearly knew who he was, so I asked. His name was David. He was born and bred in San Francisco, in a family dedicated to human rights activism. His parents wrote books and lectured, and his brother worked with special needs children. Most recently, David had been an aide to the mayor. He had left to run this campaign, a citywide initiative for policies to boost solar energy—back when no one had heard of solar panels. He spoke of solar technology as though it would, without a doubt, save our planet.

"Are you an environmentalist?" he asked me after his speech. He had come over to greet the folks I was talking to and introduced himself to me.

"I'm a doctor," I said.

"Great! We always need good doctors."

"This campaign…it's very inspiring. You're going for some big changes."

"Thanks for being a part of it." An earnest, open-mouthed smile spread across his face. We spoke for a few more minutes. Then he asked for my phone number.

"Um, just so it's clear…" I said, playing with the silver chain around my neck, the ring hidden from view. "I'm dating, but not *really* dating, if you know what I mean."

He was unfazed. "Okay, let's call it 'just having a good time.'"

A week later, I arrived at his place, the upper flat of a classic Victorian overlooking Dolores Park. His view was of a panoramic cityscape, the kind in postcards, and I paused to take it in. The Mission District was sunnier and livelier than my side of town, ornate murals adorning the buildings and Latin dance music filling the streets, couples strolling the sidewalks. A streetcar pulled to the corner, screeched to a halt, and let out a group of giggling girls.

David opened the door with his hair still damp. When he smiled, his sea-blue eyes lit up. I gave him a hug and asked if we could explore the neighborhood. He suggested we walk to Dolores Park Cafe. As we traipsed downhill, his corduroys swished with each long stride. He was much taller than me, and I found myself skipping to keep up.

"Once upon a time," he said, "there was a yellow dog, a boy, and a girl." He nudged me.

"Ah," I said, realizing the next thread was mine. "They walked by a lagoon and there was a noise that frightened them."

"When they listened more closely, it turned out to be laughter."

"But the boy wandered away and they got separated."

We arrived at the café before we finished. Dining on the patio, I talked about my passions—Russian literature, Carl Jung, and a good philosophical discussion. David talked about his—the Supreme Court, World War II, and the San Francisco 49ers. When we compared time-lines of our adult lives, during the seven years I was in medical training, he spent a year in the Bay Area guiding river rafting trips for at-risk youth; a year in a South African township teaching in a program Nelson Mandela had started; two years in Boston studying for a master's in public policy; a summer interning in the Clinton White House; then two years working for San Francisco mayor Willie Brown.

"You've had an incredible life," I said. "What were the most memo-rable experiences?"

"Playing basketball."

I nudged him. "I'm serious."

"I am, too," he laughed. "Wherever I am in the world, I can sniff out a pick-up game of hoops. Believe it or not, I packed a basketball when I went to South Africa, where no one had ever played. I used it to teach cooperation and other life skills. And as a bonus, I got to play every day." He picked at the crumbs on his plate. "But I wanna hear about you. Why'd you become a doctor?"

"The answer's in here somewhere." I reached into my shoulder bag and pulled out a book, the French Renaissance philosopher Michel de Montaigne's essays on the twenty rules for living. I read aloud, "*Pay attention. Be born. Read a lot....*"

"And here I was thinking you'd say you wanted to help people."

"That, too, of course. One of Montaigne's rules is to survive love and loss. Let's just say I don't do well with either. Or with uncertainty. Medicine seemed like the best place to address my fears." I toyed with my fork. "Isn't that what drives us—our fears more than our passions?"

"I think I'm more driven by passion."

"Of course you are," I said, chuckling. "I suppose I could lighten up a bit."

"Don't." He touched my hand. "I love how deeply you live."

Feeling at ease, I went into how my evangelical upbringing influenced my choice. David spoke of his childhood, too. His mother was a sociologist and his father a historian, both academics. He was raised with human rights as the closest thing to religion. With no real exposure to spirituality, he was eager for conversations about it; he just needed someone to ask the questions he didn't know to ask. By the time we walked to my car, I was laughing like I hadn't since Kurt died. A man of his word, David didn't try to kiss me. I hugged him good night.

Over the coming months, David invited me to group events. A talk on globalization by former president Bill Clinton. A political fund-raiser where we met actor Warren Beatty. A visit to the Tactile Dome at the Exploratorium museum. David's circle of friends and family gave me an instant community, an extensive and colorful one. Nicknamed "Mr. Sociable" by his parents, he seemingly kept in touch with his entire global network, hosting gatherings in his flat, from fund-raisers for friends running for city council to "idea brunches," where people brought a breakfast dish and an idea to make the world better (my favorites were a shag onesie so babies could mop the floor as they crawled, and a laundromat-gym where people on exercise bikes powered their own washers, with extra spin cycles for the avid cyclist).

We also spent time one-on-one. He picked me up after work one Tuesday, his car packed with sleeping bags, gear, food, and Happy the dog. He drove us an hour north to the Point Reyes National Seashore, where we camped out under the stars. The next morning, we woke before dawn, had breakfast, then he dropped me off for a regular day at the clinic. Another time, he showed up at my house at ten p.m., a double kayak strapped to the top of his car, and drove us to Sausalito, where we paddled in the moonlight, accompanied by a pair of sea lions. Our eyes locked. We smiled, kept things platonic, and continued paddling.

"How do you live like this?" I asked.

"Like what?"

"Like life is so good all the time."

He looked at me, confused.

"Hanging out with you..."—I searched for the right analogy—"...reminds me of those LIFE IS GOOD T-shirts, the ones with the smiley faces on them. You know what I'm talking about?"

He nodded, but still looked confused.

"I'm not complaining. But I never fully trusted that motto. It's too simplistic. It's like Newton's Third Law: For every action, there's an equal and opposite reaction."

"And your point is...?"

"My point is...just when you think things are good, something hard follows."

Our kayaks had drifted so that David's face was hidden by shadows. I assumed from his silence that I wasn't making sense to him. "I was engaged before. His name was Kurt. He died in a car accident two years ago."

David was quiet. I couldn't see him clearly, and the silence felt awkward. "I'm sorry."

"For what? I'm the one who's sorry. I'm shocked. I had no—"

"Sorry for not telling you sooner, sorry for bringing you down, sorry for complicating things. I wasn't looking to date—"

"Technically, we're not dating."

My eyes widened. "Just because we haven't kissed or had sex?" I shook my head, thinking, *Right, as if experiences can be defined like that.* But in that moment, I realized David was doing what I had so often tried to do: to control life's variables and make them neater than they actually were.

We drove back to my place and talked about Kurt all night. My housemates came home, said hello, then good night. David and I dozed on and off on the couch. In the wee hours of the morning, I took out the shoebox of Kurt's things. Lying in David's arms, I selected certain letters to read aloud. I felt lighter, and David felt deepened by the conversation. Then we kissed. We kissed until the first bright rays broke through the blinds.

To get ready for work, I drank a cup of coffee, washed my face, and changed into a blouse and skirt. In the bathroom mirror, I twirled my necklace—Kurt's ring—then took it off and tucked it away in Kurt's shoebox, leaving the cover off to give his spirit some air. "I love you," I whispered to the shoebox, "and I love him."

David and I wed the following spring.

The inscription on our wedding bands: *Love endures all things.*

After the wedding, I quit my job. I had never made such an impulsive decision before, but David had that effect on me. Wrapping up another intense campaign, he had an opportunity to take a six-month leave and proposed that we travel abroad. Now was the time, he said. We didn't have children, we had the rest of our lives to focus on our careers…why the heck not?

My heart leaped. Why *not?* This was a question I rarely asked. David pushed it further. "Let's travel without an itinerary." No plan? It was a bold new philosophy: have more fun, trust the world to take care of us, and let life unfold. I must have been ready, because it took me all of ten minutes to agree, and once I did, I was all in. We bought an RTW (Round the World) flexible ticket and packed backpacks with only our barest essentials. Letting go of all practicalities, I proposed that New Zealand be our first stop, having just watched *The Lord of the Rings* trilogy. We didn't find any hobbits, but we encountered a lot of sheep, climbed a glacier, and did some spelunking in caves.

From there, we cast emails far and wide, to friends and family who might want to host two wandering Americans, and received more invitations than we could accept. After New Zealand, we set off for the red rock of Australia, then the islands of the South Pacific, the savannas of South Africa, and the shores of Senegal. At the end of six months, David had to return to his job in San Francisco. But I had quit mine.

"I'd like to travel for one more month, solo," I said, wanting to go to China. My parents had moved to Beijing from Texas during my medical training, and it was time to pay them a visit. I had also heard that Doctors Without Borders was establishing an HIV/AIDS clinic in the countryside there, and wanted to participate.

The experience in the Chinese farming community affected me deeply. The families had been devastated by contaminated blood donation practices, and of the three generations that were typically living under one roof, the middle generation was largely sick or dying. Our medical team made farm calls and treated patients who otherwise had no access to care. The families treated us to meals of homegrown vegetables as we discussed treatment plans. In addition to the drugs we provided, the families used folk remedies like herbs when nothing else helped their eczema and seborrhea. Some cooked freshwater eels, purported to boost the immune system. I wrote daily emails to David on how differently medicine was done here—the slower pace, the team effort, the collaboration with patients, the self-care—and all of it with extremely limited resources. I knew when I returned that I wanted to work with marginalized communities. Those that had been left behind.

I returned to San Francisco, reinvigorated. David had dinner waiting for me. I put on some Chopin piano music and we ate, exchanged stories, made love, then exchanged more stories. I told him I would look for a job here, but hoped we could go abroad again when the timing was right.

"I'm all for it," he said, tickling me. "You're less conventional than you appear."

I grabbed his arms and tickled him back. Making up for lost time, we made love again, this time to Debussy.

The canvas of my life was splattered with vibrant reds, oranges, and greens. As David fell into a gentle snore, I lay there reflecting, *Life is good.*

FOUR

2004

Our wedding and travels over, I settled into David's flat in the Mission District. His flat, one of several row houses, had a decent-size bedroom, a small bathroom, a small living area, and a small kitchen. By San Francisco standards, it was ample space for two. We were on the upper level, complete with a "fainting room," a miniature room at the top of old Victorian buildings, designed for women to recuperate from their tight corsets. The floor-to-ceiling bay windows provided a greater spaciousness. From Dolores Park below, we could always hear something going on: a political rally, the mime troupe, or parades by the Sisters of Perpetual Indulgence.

David's friend Juan Carlos lived in the flat below us. He was a teacher-turned-acupuncture student. I had never known anyone quite like him. A lifelong vegetarian, he believed in a sustainable and compassionate world. He loathed waste in any form, got around by bike, and bought his clothes secondhand. The trash he generated might fill a small bag in a month. When I moved in, he was in the middle of an experiment of living without electricity for six months, including no heat or refrigeration.

I was grateful to have this community, but this setup was a big adjustment for me. San Francisco still felt new. Moving into David's place in David's city with David's good friend below and David's family close by, I had a hard time feeling like this life was mine. When Juan Carlos popped upstairs to grab us for soccer or frisbee in the park, or David's other friends dropped by with regularity, I felt a self-imposed expectation to connect with everyone, now, and deeply. Life was moving so fast. I had the impression of skipping along to keep up with David's long strides.

Sometimes I hopped the streetcar back to the foggy side of the city and caught up with my old roommates. Sometimes I visited Ocean Beach or Golden Gate Park, passing an hour or two under a blanket in the fog, with a book like Dostoevsky's *The Brothers Karamazov* or Vonnegut's *Cat's Cradle* in my lap and a sushi roll in my hand. My MDR—minimum daily requirement—of solitude and time in nature was increasing.

I took a new job at the county hospital a mile and a half from our house. Not only could I walk to work, my position was at the urgent care center, which meant no more on-call or night shifts. To top it off, appointments were allotted thirty whole minutes. My patients were made up of people living with HIV/AIDS, refugees, homeless families, and the working uninsured. When I heard their stories, I realized how little I knew about real suffering. One patient complained of chronic neck pain. When I asked about her mattress, she admitted that she didn't have one. She slept in her car, had for twenty years, and had raised two children in it. Another patient complained of an ingrown toenail that was causing him terrible pain. When I examined his feet, both were blistered, oozy, and putrid. Living on the streets, he was so used to the general poor condition of his feet that his only concern that day—he kept his chief complaints to one—was his toenail. Some days I left the clinic in tears.

David continued to build a nonprofit organization, promoting renewable energy policies for cities and states across the country. With his partner, he fought to shut down dirty power plants and worked for environmental justice, gaining the attention of foundations and getting enough donations to hire a third person.

In the evenings, we would debrief each other about our workdays. As we lay on the couch together, David would massage my feet and pop the knuckles on my toes, one by one. Sometimes our ritual involved chocolate ice cream and bonbons. His mouth full, David would say how he envied the immediate successes I experienced in the clinic. I would say how I envied his large-scale impacts.

I adored our one-on-one time. The exchange of ideas, the humor, and the sex. Sex was how we wound down our days, and often how we started them, too. Just after my thirty-third birthday, we agreed it was time "to pull the goalie," as David put it—to stop my birth control pills. I wasn't sure I was ready for motherhood, but I knew that complications increased with age, and I was just a couple of years shy of AMA, or advanced maternal age. With the goalie pulled, my periods remained regular and my weight dropped a couple pounds, but the greatest change was my libido. It turned out being unguarded—tempting fate—evoked a fear-laced excitement. So the pleasure of sex, if I could ascribe it a color, turned from orange to raging crimson.

I missed my period the very next month. I peed on a stick, and David and I waited five long minutes. One pink line appeared. Then two! It was positive! We jumped up and down with the same fear-laced excitement that had invited this baby in. How was it possible that the fusion of David's chromosomes and protoplasm with mine had created a little being we could hold in our arms in less than a year's time? The pregnancy felt abstract until my first obstetrics visit, when the doctor squirted lubricating jelly on my belly and rolled the ultrasound probe around. I heard it first—a faint heartbeat, *lub-dub, lub-dub,* humming along at twice the rate as mine. Then I saw it—a shadow no bigger than a bonbon, surrounded by a halo of white, with a flickering spark in the middle. This was realer than real.

My belly grew. I did prenatal yoga twice a week. I walked three miles round-trip, to and from work, every day. Toward the end of the pregnancy, my hands and tendons ached—carpal tunnel syndrome from fluid retention—but the nine months passed swiftly. Come the following summer, baby Rosa joined our family.

From the moment we got home from the hospital, I sunk into our couch and put her tiny lips to my breast and began a love affair of a whole new kind. I would watch her suckle and sleep for hours. I would stroke her heels, which were supple like lambskin. A dormant part of my heart seemed to awaken. My sense of self now included this fascinating little being. We were a coordinated, symbiotic unit, my mind attuned to her different cries; my body producing breastmilk with the perfect proportions of fatty acids, proteins, and sugars, and releasing the right hormones at the right time, synchronized with her feeding schedule. And none of this required any medical interventions or special degrees. It felt like a superpower.

For the first three months, I took maternity leave. David took a week off, then resumed his long work hours. I saw domestic duties as my job and took it upon myself to do all the feedings, day and night, and the lion's share of the housework. Nurse the baby. Change her diaper. Run a load of laundry. Dry. Fold. Nurse again. Put her down for a nap. Tidy up. Sweep. Baby's awake. Nurse again. Shop. Cook. Do the dishes. Pump breastmilk. Store. Wash bottles. Nurse again. Give baby a bath. Wait, the laundry basket's full again? With every chore taking twice as long with a baby to tend to, and a body that was recovering, I was more exhausted now than in residency. At least then, I wasn't on call twenty-four seven.

After the blur of the first month, I let a lot of things go. The laundry basket would overflow. The dishes often piled up. Mostly, I wanted to enjoy my time with Rosa. I developed a sweet morning routine with her. After she nursed, I would strap her into a baby carrier and take a morning stroll. Down the hill to Tartine Bakery for an almond croissant, then to Bi-Rite Market for some gouda or feta for the house, then to my favorite bench in Dolores Park, where we would watch dogs running around on the hill. As Rosa grew increasingly aware of the world beyond her fingers and toes, our stays at the park grew longer. Right about the time she began to smile, I was scheduled to return to work.

I went back three days a week, but missed Rosa when I was there. David's parents, who lived a mile away from us, would take care of her. Writers by profession, they could adjust their schedules, and the arrangement thrilled them. We also hired a Chinese woman to help two mornings a week, mostly with housework. We called her He Ayi, or Ayi ("Auntie") for short. She was in her sixties, and as strong as an ox. Since she was older and Chinese, I fell into the custom of deferring to her. Sometimes I spoke my mind, but unless I had a strong preference for how something was to be done, I let her do it her way. David found it hard to relate to Ayi's stoic pragmatism, but I was totally comfortable, having grown up with it. In many ways, she reminded me of my mother. Ayi's approval of how we kept our house—her approval of me—mattered a great deal.

"Now that I'm back at work," I said, handing David the dish sponge, "things at home will have to change."

"But that's why we hired Ayi, isn't it?"

"Oh, she'll be a huge help. But she's only here six hours a week. Ultimately, this is *our* home, and you and I will need to split things fifty-fifty."

"Sure, absolutely," he said. "I can do that."

But before we settled into parenthood and work, life displaced me from *here* to *there*.

I was walking uphill from Dolores Park one morning, with Rosa strapped to my chest in a carrier. Then for a second, I lost my breath. I stopped and inhaled deeply, noticing a faint flutter in my chest. *A muscle twitch?* I wondered. But it continued, and I felt a little winded, even just standing there resting. So I cut through the grass, dashed home, and went to the fainting room at the top of the stairs. On the black swivel chair, I unstrapped Rosa and waited for the flutter to pass. Moments later, I felt myself again and got dressed for work. The day was otherwise ordinary.

That night, I felt like I was coming down with a cold. A malaise in the shoulders, a slight chill. My throat was sore, but the soreness was on the outside. I checked my lymph nodes for lumps and swelling. Nothing. So I took two tablets of ibuprofen.

David was in bed, reading *The New Yorker*. He called me over to look at the cartoon contest in the back, but I wasn't interested. He looked disappointed, as this had been an activity we enjoyed together. "Help me come up with something witty," he said. "You're so much better at it than I am."

"But she needs to be tipped off for the night," I said, turning to Rosa. She was lying quietly in a bassinet next to our bed. I picked her up and nursed her in the rocking chair, holding her close and rubbing her heels until she fell asleep. I held her against my chest for a while longer, then returned her to the bassinet.

As I undressed for bed, David got up behind me and turned my body forty-five degrees. "Look," he said, pointing to my bare contours. In the full-length mirror, my muscles appeared sunken, as if a sculptor had molded them concave instead of convex. "Are you eating enough?"

"A ton," I said, studying my body in the mirror. I was eating four or five meals a day, with hearty snacks in between, including extra helpings of ice cream. I figured it must have been the effects of breastfeeding. Nursing mothers needed five hundred extra calories or more a day, and my metabolism was fast to begin with. Chalking up my strange symptoms to postpartum stuff, I went to the kitchen and made myself a turkey sandwich.

When I returned to the bedroom, David was waiting for me in bed. Between my patients, the baby, and David, I felt stretched like a worn-out rubber band, less and less able to bounce back. Quiet time had become scarce, far below my MDR, and I was craving some now. What's more, my sex drive had plummeted. I knew that breastfeeding hormones could suppress sex hormones, but I hadn't realized how much. Pleasure was reduced to localized tingles, and when David touched me, my thoughts often drifted to Rosa. She was the one I longed to be skin-to-skin with.

This was a huge change for our marriage. So when David stroked my back that night, I didn't say no. I wanted to show that I still loved him. I turned on the CD player and let him pick the music. Manu Chao—alternative reggae in Spanish. As we made love to the world beat, I tried to lose myself, but couldn't.

In the coming weeks, a paradox of symptoms erupted: pimples broke out on my forehead and hot flashes surged through my body, as though puberty and menopause had hit at once. I was revved up and lethargic, sharp and forgetful, tired and unable to sleep. The insomnia was the worst symptom. Night after night, I lay wide awake.

As my sleeplessness grew, a distance came between David and me. Watching his deep breaths and hearing his whistling nose, I envied, then resented, the ease with which he slept. I was nursing, so I didn't want any sleep medicine, even those deemed safe for breastfeeding mothers. By morning, I would look in the mirror and see a Gorgon with wild hair and dark circles under her eyes. If I started to worry about the effects of sleep deprivation, I would redirect my attention to the baby and get myself to work. At the clinic, if my heart fluttered intermittently or my body burned up like a furnace, I would take a quick break, collect myself, then move on to the next patient.

On the home front, normalcy was harder to maintain. I often came home to dirty clothes in the hamper or dishes piled in the sink. More than a few times, I lashed out at David: Why aren't you helping with the housework? What about the nighttime feeds? The shopping? The cooking? He would look genuinely puzzled. Only after I yelled would he get off the couch and help. And for every time I yelled out loud, I must have yelled in my mind fifty times.

One day, David tried to broach this tension. We were eating sandwiches on the back deck. The sun was shining. Rosa was in a baby hammock, dangling between the doorframe.

"Have you been feeling okay?" he asked.

I shrugged my shoulders, not wanting to ruin the beautiful day.

"I feel like I've been walking on eggshells," he continued.

"Look," I said. I knew what he was talking about. "I've had to rearrange my whole life around motherhood, while your life has largely stayed the same. That was fine when I was on maternity leave, but now I'm working again, and you don't seem to notice that I'm busy, too. You never chip in. It's like I'm invisible until I make some noise."

He paused, then said, "I'm worried you're not getting enough sleep."

"I would get more sleep if you helped with the night feeds."

"But night feeds or not," he said, mouth full, "you can't sleep, right?"

Rage was foaming in my throat, like bubbles ready to burst. I restrained it with all I had. "Why are you bringing up my sleep? I'm talking about *your* need to step up. Stop changing the subject."

"I just know how I feel when I don't get enough sleep. Maybe it's making you more irritable."

You're what's making me irritable, I yelled inside my mind. I mashed a fallen plum on the deck with my shoe. The simple act was so satisfying I mashed a few more, rubbing the pulp deep into the cracks between the wooden planks.

"Hey," he blurted, "what are you doing that for?"

"What does it matter? I'm the one who ends up cleaning everything anyhow."

He stood up.

"Where are you going?" I asked.

"To play some basketball."

"Basketball?"

"You're confusing me too much."

The truth is, I was confusing me, too. What was this volatility—postpartum hormones? Motherhood? Sheer fatigue? Moodiness was new to me, hadn't touched me even in residency, when I was over-worked and sleep-deprived. Yet I couldn't admit this to David. I needed him to step up with the day-to-day responsibilities, which were a real and separate issue. What I hadn't fully grasped at the time was that the more disordered I became on the inside, the more order I needed around me, as though the inner and outer were weighing against one another on a precarious scale, trying to keep me sane.

Once he was gone, I mashed another plum on the deck.

The following week was routine at the clinic. Until the last patient on Friday. She was in her thirties, a single mother of three, working two jobs. I couldn't imagine how she was still standing. It didn't surprise me that her chief complaint was the dreaded "fatigue." She needed a long, all-expenses-paid holiday.

"I've been feeling awful for a few weeks," she said, her eyes tearing up. "I have so much to do, kids to take care of, bills to pay…"

I took a thorough history: heart palpitations, insomnia, shortness of breath. I followed with a thorough physical: resting heart rate elevated, reflexes jumpy, ten pounds below her usual weight.

"You've got all the signs of hyperthyroidism," I said. She was a textbook case of an overactive thyroid gland. A sharp pain gripped my gut. The flutter in my chest, the soreness on my neck, the muscle wasting, the moods—*I* was a textbook case, too.

FIVE

2005

I hadn't ever conceived of having a health condition, much less one of the thyroid. Thyroid conditions are usually chronic, meaning they don't resolve on their own, like the flu or a sprained ankle, and they tend to progress or relapse. At thirty-four, I still had the illusion of youthful invincibility. But it was more than that. I also had the illusion of doctorhood—I imagined my knowledge of diseases would provide an immunity against them. My patients were *there* (in illness) and I was *here* (in wellness). Or was supposed to be.

Once I realized that might not be the case, I did my best to control the variables in my favor. I became obsessed with getting a diagnosis. My degree offered me huge advantages. Instead of waiting for an appointment, then waiting for labs to return, then waiting another day or two to get the call, and only then getting to see a specialist, I ordered my own labs. And three days later, my thyroid hormones came back sky-high.

I was angry. I was relieved.

The thyroid gland is a bowtie-shaped gland in the front of the neck. When it's working properly, it doesn't get much notice. Like air traffic control, its significance is underrated until it's off-kilter. Mine was either producing or releasing too much thyroid hormone, which controls metabolism; and metabolism is much more than simply weight gain or loss. It's the fundamental process of transforming food into energy, occurring in every cell of the body. My thyroid hormones were telling my cells to use, produce, and recycle energy too fast. This gave me the felt experience of failing to keep up with my own inner workings. The mnemonic I had learned in medical school summed it up. THYROIDISM: Tremor, Heart palpitations, Yawning, Restlessness, Oligomenorrhea (reduced menstrual cycles), Intolerance to heat,

<u>D</u>iarrhea, <u>I</u>rritability, <u>S</u>weating, <u>M</u>uscle wasting. This was hardly the news I wanted. But naming it gave me information, and information was power.

Labs in hand, I went to see a top-notch endocrinologist who focused on thyroid disorders. He had a grandfatherly air that reminded me of my mentor, Dr. Eisenberg. His snow-white hair matched his immaculate doctor's coat. Underneath, he wore a pressed shirt, a two-tone bowtie, and a tweed vest. He smelled either like a closet of woolly sweaters or an antique store—I couldn't tell which—but I liked it.

"So you're an internist," he said, articulating each word.

"Yes," I said, smiling. I felt like I was back in residency, meeting an attending doctor.

He took a comprehensive history.

Past medical history? None.

Family history? Diabetes and hypertension, otherwise unremarkable.

Past surgical history? None.

Social history? No drugs or tobacco or alcohol.

Next, he began the physical exam by inserting a thermometer into my ear, and something in me shifted. My colleague-to-colleague confidence turned into a stark awareness of my nakedness under the thin paper gown, and I wondered how in the world I had ended up on the wrong side of the bedside. Say *ahhh*, he said. *Ahhh.* Again. *Ahhh.* I tried to relax and be a good patient.

My temperature was 99 degrees Fahrenheit. *Mild hyperthermia* (body temperature too hot). Resting heart rate in the 90s. *Tachycardia* (rapid heart rate). *Blood pressure 110/70* (normal). He asked me to look up and down. *No evidence of eye involvement* (one form of hyperthyroidism—Graves' Disease—can result in bulging eyes). He palpated my throat, asked me to swallow, and put his stethoscope over my thyroid. *No goiter, bruits, nodules, or lymph nodes* (thyroid not enlarged, no bumps, no swollen glands). He listened to my heart and lungs. *Normal rhythm, equal breath sounds, no wheezes or rales.* He tapped my reflexes, checked for tremors, and pressed my ankles. *Hyperreflexic, tremulous, no edema* (reflexes too brisk, fingers shaky, but no swelling in the legs or feet).

"You're clearly hyperthyroid," he said. "Most likely, it's postpartum thyroiditis. But your labs are a little unusual. We ought to rule out other kinds of hyperthyroidism."

"What do you recommend?"

"A thyroid scan. It's pretty straightforward. Shouldn't disrupt your life too much. In and out."

"You mean a nuclear scan?"

"Yes."

I had ordered this same test on many patients of my own. But on the receiving end, the word *nuclear* sounded different. Dangerous, to be specific. Still early in my career, I hadn't seen any cases of postpartum thyroid disease, and I knew that he was the expert. His certainty gave me hope; and with my moods and sleep a mess and my thinking less clear, I told myself I didn't have to worry. I thanked him and took his requisition in hand.

I returned to the hospital for my scan a few days later. A tech with platinum hair checked me in, then took me to the back room, where he presented me with a red and yellow capsule on a plate. This was radioactive iodine, a tracer taken up by the thyroid. It was low-dose radiation. Useful, but also a poison.

He brought the plate closer. "Pretend it's a vitamin."

It's a necessary test, I told myself, and swallowed it with a glass of water.

"Come back tomorrow, same time," he said. "I'll take some additional images, and then you'll be done."

As I walked out, multiple posters around the room read CAUTION—RADIOACTIVE MATERIALS. And it dawned on me, I was oozing radioactivity! It hadn't occurred to me that my radiation might affect others. No one had mentioned it—not my endocrinologist, nor the tech.

"I'm confused," I said to the tech, trying to hide my anger. "I have a baby. Am I safe to hold her?"

"Hmm, you know, we recommend patients self-quarantine for a week, but that's only when we use much higher doses of radiation." He scratched his head. "The dose you got was much smaller. Shouldn't be much of a problem."

My stomach sunk. I didn't want to expose Rosa to anything, and I realized it was up to me to figure things out. I drove home, rage foaming in my throat. How could radioactive tests be handled so casually? Why was it up to me to ask about toxicity? Did my endocrinologist assume I knew because I was a doctor? Did he even think that I might be nursing my baby? I had more pressing issues right now. During the two hours I was at the hospital, my breasts had become engorged. *My breastmilk!* I thought. *It* was radioactive, too!

I pulled over to the curb. Trying to contain my emotions, I made some phone calls. Between David, his parents, Juan Carlos, Ayi, and baby formula, I pieced together a plan. By the end, I was toxic, all right—with fury.

At home, I got on my laptop to do some research. As I was searching for radioactivity, I came across the risks of thyroid scans and other tests involving radiation, like CT and PET scans. Sure, they were useful to diagnose, treat, stage a disease, and track the response to a treatment. But there were long-term side-effects I hadn't known. The greater the radiation exposure, the greater the risk of cancer over a person's lifetime. There were other complications, too. Thyroid scans increased the risk, ironically, of hypothyroidism. Since these health effects might not develop for years or decades, the harm was difficult to measure. Not surprisingly, surveys showed that less than half of doctors ordering the tests knew about these risks.

As for radioactive iodine-123, the particular tracer I had taken, the half-life was 13.22 hours. This meant half the amount would remain in my body after 13.22 hours, then half of the remaining amount would be left after the next 13.22 hours, and so on. If I did my calculations right, after three weeks, the remains would be roughly 3.687723^{-11}—or whatever that number translates to, a billionth of the tracer? Close enough to zero, I thought. So for the next three weeks, I pumped and discarded my breast milk at a makeshift pumping station in the garage. Several times a day, I would sit under a flickering lightbulb and breathe in mildew and gasoline fumes while a monotonous *swish, swish* tugged on my breasts. I could never get used to the last part—pouring my milk into large plastic buckets, then later down the drain. Because my maternal confidence was in that milk.

A week after my scan, I returned to the clinic to discuss my results. My original grandfatherly endocrinologist was away, so a different doctor showed me my scan. A normal thyroid would appear as two black thumbprints on a white screen. Mine was washed out, with faint dots scattered throughout. My diagnosis: postpartum thyroiditis.

"Is there anything I can do?"

"Not much," he said. "Mostly, the thyroiditis just needs to run its course. You can try a medication for your palpitations. But the good news is that most cases resolve within a year."

Gathering my things, I knew I should be grateful. But really I wanted to wind the clock back a few weeks and not have to deal with this at all.

"Just out of curiosity," he said, "why'd he"—the endocrinologist—"recommend the radioactive scan?"

I cocked my head. "I don't understand."

"I was just wondering what his thought process was. Because I wouldn't have chosen a nuclear scan, especially for a postpartum case. The scan has given you a definitive diagnosis, but an ultrasound could have been helpful without exposing you to radiation."

I was incredulous. "You mean, I could have done an ultrasound instead?"

"Or you could have skipped the imaging all together and just waited to see how your course unfolded."

"Good to know. Thank you, Doctor."

On the bus ride home, I sat in the back, staring out the window, confused as to what I was feeling, scanning the sidewalk for anyone else to blame—the teenager in her headphones, a fluffy dog on the sidewalk—but I kept coming back to me. I should have known better, and I was disgusted with myself.

Back at home, I slumped into a corner in a daze.

David waved, trying to get my attention. "So what's the diagnosis?"

"Postpartum thyroiditis," I mumbled.

"And—?"

I couldn't handle a discussion about it. I couldn't shake the vision of all those buckets of tainted breastmilk. In trying to think about something else, my eyes locked on the dishes in the sink and the crumbs on the floor. "Why do I *always* have to ask you to help out?" I pointed to the sink. "This is *our* house, not *mine* to clean."

"Whoa, babe, calm down. It doesn't have to be perfect all the time. And I'll get to it later."

"I don't want perfection!" I yelled, swiping a lint ball from the corner. "Just some balance and equality! And some initiative on your part!"

"This anger doesn't sound like you." He was tiptoeing with his words. "I don't think this is you talking. It's your hormones."

I spotted another lint ball and smacked it. "I *am* my fucking hormones!" I stormed out back, where the air was crisp, the sun was yellow, and the wind was still.

Fifteen minutes must have passed when David brought out a tray of fresh-squeezed lemonade. "Can we try this again? I want to hear how things went today. Help me understand what *thyroiditis* means."

Appreciating the peace gesture, I opted to try again, describing my situation with a dose of detachment, even adding a touch of magic to make up for my earlier outburst: "It's...it's like my immune system is a dragon."

I made up a story about a dragon (my immune system) that once fended off invaders from the kingdom (my body). These invaders were wicked creatures: viruses, bacteria, and parasites. But the dragon was given confusing messages (my shifting postpartum hormones), and it started breathing fire (inflammation) at the kingdom itself, or at least part of it (my thyroid). The fire didn't self-extinguish as it was supposed to. So the singed walls of the kingdom (the thyroid cells) began to crumble, releasing their goods from storage (thyroid hormones). And the overflow of stored goods wreaked more havoc on the kingdom as a whole (other parts of my body).

By the end of my story, I was sufficiently cooled off. I took a few sips of lemonade and thanked David for it.

"Let me make sure I understand you correctly," he said. "Your body's attacking itself?"

I nodded.

"But why'd you get this in the first place?"

"No one really knows. Why and when autoimmunity turns on is rather murky. Female hormones definitely play a role. It's common after pregnancy and around menopause. Five to seven percent of women get this after they have a baby. The biggest risk for thyroiditis is family history."

"I didn't know this ran in your family," David said.

"It doesn't."

As far as I knew, anyway.

The hyperthyroid madness lasted two months. Then my hormones—and, consequently, my metabolism—fell too low (*hypo*-thyroidism). The mnemonic from medical school was Hyp-O-thyroidism: Overweight, On a downer, On ice. Now out of gas, I lumbered around the house, cranked the heat up, and lathered myself in lotion, as my once oily, acne-prone skin had turned dry and scaly. Instead of rage bubbles in my throat, I felt little emotion at all. The canvas of my life turned into a grayish-green veil, as if creating a distance between others and me. I tried to explain it to David one night when he found me in bed, sweatpants on, earplugs in, reading.

"I feel detached, almost dissociated, from everyone else. Novels are the only things that make me feel less alone. Like the stories have an authenticity I can't otherwise connect to in reality. Maybe it's that I feel alone—"

"I can help you feel less alone," he said, drawing the covers off me.

"I'm cold," I said, drawing them back up.

"*I'll* warm you up."

"Sorry, not tonight."

David sighed and grabbed a *Rolling Stone* magazine. I watched as he climbed into bed. He looked like a stranger. The distance between us felt enormous.

I started taking a medication called levothyroxine, a synthetic thyroid hormone, to bring my levels into the normal range. I also resorted to splashing my face with cold water, pinching myself, and doing jumping jacks to pump up enough momentum to get myself to work. At the clinic, I often treated patients with hypothyroidism or suspected hypothyroidism. It was inevitable, since more than twenty million Americans had a thyroid disorder. When these patients reported persistent symptoms despite adequate blood levels of thyroid hormone, I had nothing to offer. Rx: pinch yourself, do jumping jacks? I missed the clear difference that I used to make in my patients' lives. Treating acute conditions or acute exacerbations of chronic conditions in the hospital was a totally different strategy than managing chronic conditions for long-term well-being. Between appointments, as I sat in the charting room trying to overcome the inertia in my body, I felt like a closeted sufferer unable to "come out." Still, I believed in medicine as I had been taught. The tests were objective. They had the final word.

I powered through my symptoms, working three days a week, fulfilling domestic duties, and trying to keep up with David's very active life. Gradually, I seemed to adjust better to my condition, though I wasn't sure why. Perhaps my body had adjusted to the thyroid medication. Perhaps the inflammation from the autoimmune response was diminishing. Perhaps I was more fully recovered from pregnancy and childbirth. Perhaps my mind-over-matter strategies were working. Or perhaps it was a combination of all those factors. In this relatively steady state, I called my parents, sister, and brothers, to update them on my health. And to give them a warning.

"I'm the sentinel case," I said. "We now have a family history of auto-immune thyroid disease, which means you're at increased risk, too."

"What can we do about it?" my parents asked.

"Um…" I said, thinking. *Was* there anything they could do? Could their risk be reduced? Was it just a matter of watchful waiting and hoping they were spared? I didn't know, and I didn't handle I-don't-know very well.

Trying to reassert my expertise, I replied, "Stay healthy. Eat well, and exercise."

A few months later, my younger brother, who was in Texas, experienced symptoms consistent with hyperthyroidism and was diagnosed with Graves' disease. My sister, a year later, and my father, a few years later, both living in China, would develop Hashimoto's, an autoimmune form of *hypo*thyroidism. I didn't understand it beyond genes, but I would later learn about multiple factors that might have contributed to this family epidemic. And as Rosa approached her first birthday and crawled into forbidden spaces, pulled herself up against the furniture, and, soon thereafter, tottered on her own two feet, I worried about *her* risk of developing autoimmune thyroid disease. My parents' question, What can we do about it?, became a seed planted in my mind. My family history was now far from "unremarkable."

Also around this time, the thyroid doctor was recommending that I taper off my thyroid medication, to see if my numbers would normal-ize. I did. Off medication, my numbers stayed in the normal range.

"Hallelujah!" David cheered. "So, which one was worse, hyper- or hypo-?"

"Both," I said.

Despite the numbers, I didn't feel like *me*. My sleep remained poor, my energy diminished. I was fully functional, though. And since the thyroiditis had started so soon after Rosa's birth, I could never fully sort out which parts were motherhood-related and which were thyroid-related. Not knowing what "normal" was, in essence, I considered myself cured.

SIX

2007

The following spring, my body seemed to be sorting itself out. My energy was up a notch, and some weekends I could go jogging or rollerblading in Golden Gate Park while pushing Rosa in a stroller. I was no longer nursing Rosa, which, in theory, meant my sex hormones would return to pre-pregnancy levels. While my libido didn't return with vigor, I had more space to pay attention to emotional and physical intimacy. If irritations arose with David, I made a concerted effort to restrain my outbursts and respond with affection. If opportunities to enjoy our shared interests arose, I took them—good food and adventurous travel above all. Traveling always brought out the best in our relationship, and I thought a change in scenery might reboot our marriage. So one night, I proposed a family trip.

"What do you think about Beijing?" I said. I was now a few years overdue in visiting my parents.

"I'd love to see your folks," David said. "But Beijing isn't my idea of a vacation. It's so polluted and congested."

"I know. But my parents have been dying to show us around and to introduce Rosa to the sights."

"She's two years old. How much will she remember?"

"It's the gesture." I nudged him. "Besides, I'd like to see my mom. Now that I'm a mother, I've got something in common with her. Maybe we'll understand each other better."

"You're still needing her approval," he said, his tone questioning.

"Not her approval," I said, fiddling with my hair. "I'd just like for us to get to know each other, adult to adult." I promised he could pick our next trip.

So in late April, we set off on a ten-day trip to Beijing.

My parents packed our days like overzealous tour guides. The Forbidden City...Tiananmen Square...open flea markets...shopping malls...ancient palaces...endless temples...meals with cousins...an orphanage...a visit to their church. Without much downtime, we didn't have any heart-to-heart talks, but my parents had a wonderful time with Rosa. She brought out in them a playful affection, which was good enough for me.

After a week in the megatropolis, David and I asked for an escape. My parents took us to the "Wild Wall," an untouched portion of the Great Wall an hour's drive away. It was a part of China I had never seen. The green mountains stretched out forever. The air was steamy, but the sky was expansive, a huge improvement on the solid gray canopy over the city. Ancient bricks held together the paths, unadorned and raw. David and I held hands as we walked, with Rosa strapped to my back in a carrier. For the first time since the thyroiditis, I felt my vitality again. As David and I climbed a watchtower and scanned the green mountains, I shouted, "I'm back to my old self!"

"How about celebrating with *jiaozi*—Chinese dumplings?" my parents asked.

We took a long bus ride back to the city center and arrived at a dumpling house that served more than a hundred varieties. Starving, the five of us waited for our food while listening to sounds in the background: porcelain teacups clinking, the air conditioner rattling, chatter filling the rooms. Finally, platter after magnificent platter of *jiaozi* appeared before our eyes: crescent moons, flower buds, ruffled squares. I sampled them all. Pork and cabbage, vegetarian delight, crab and water chestnuts, lamb and scallions.

Then came the moment that would change everything.

I was eating a twenty-mushroom special when it happened. An intense pressure shot up my spine and gripped my head, like something big and hard was forcing its way out. Seconds later, my heart rhythm snapped and thundered across my chest, and an extreme dizziness overtook me. Panicked, I lay down across the empty adjacent seat.

"Are you okay?" David said.

"I must have overdone it at the Wall," I said, trying to sound calm.

My head continued to pound. My heart thundered. Trying to be the doctor in the situation, I placed two fingers along the side of my neck to locate my carotid artery. I tried to estimate my heart rate, but it was too fast. *Common things are common,* I recited in my mind, *uncommon things are uncommon.* I scrolled through a list of common diagnoses, like dehydration and heat stroke. But drinking water didn't help, and instead seemed to make it worse. As my body continued to storm, the dizziness turned into an undertow, as though I was drowning into myself. My mind churned other possible diagnoses—an arrhythmia, a toxic mushroom, anaphylaxis, a ruptured blood vessel—with the list growing more ominous by the second. I grabbed David's hand and whisper-yelled, "Have my parents call an ambulance. *Now.*" I started to hyperventilate.

People around me were shouting in Mandarin and English, and Rosa was crying. As I continued to hyperventilate, images flashed through my mind like a movie on fast-forward: playing under my favorite cedar tree as a child, learning to drive stick shift in the red Toyota Corolla, riding on the back of my boyfriend Charles's motorcycle, playing Scrabble with Kurt, exchanging vows with David, and playing with Rosa in the sandbox. The last thing I remember was David telling my mother, "This is serious," and to never mind the leftovers. I closed my eyes, and entered a black hole where silence suffocated the ambient noise, thinking this was the end.

I woke on a gurney in a crowded emergency room in downtown Beijing. An ambulance had taken me there, and four empty IV bags hung overhead. Masses of people lined the cinder block walls, waiting to be seen by a doctor. I scanned each face, looking for David, Rosa, or my parents. But my vision was off. The room spun, as though I was peering at it through a slow-moving kaleidoscope. My muscles were off, too, clumsy and weak. My skin tingled in an unpleasant way, like electrical shocks were pricking me all over.

A young doctor arrived. In Mandarin accented by an unfamiliar dialect, he introduced himself as a resident-in-training. He began to scold me, as if I had brought this event onto myself. Seeing that I needed to assert my doctor privileges, I steadied my equilibrium enough to say *"Zai Meiguo wo shi yi sheng.* I'm a doctor in America." His tone shifted, and he offered to review my chart with me. In fact, he looked to me for guidance.

The EKG was on top, but my disequilibrium made this normally at-a-glance task a five-minute one. My heart looked okay; its rhythm must have snapped back to normal during the ambulance ride or shortly thereafter. My mind a blur, I resorted to the mnemonic for syncope (loss of consciousness), to cover all the bases. PASSOUT: Pressure—low blood pressure, dehydration; Arrhythmias—abnormal heart rhythms; Seizures; Sugar—extreme low or high blood sugars; Output—low heart output, low oxygen to tissues; Unusual causes; Transient—transient ischemic attacks, or mini-strokes. Unusual causes? I thought. What a worthless mnemonic.

I asked the doctor to order the standard emergency protocols, which he agreed to, and, given my medical history, to include a thyroid screen. As I was waiting for my results, my parents, David, and Rosa came to my bedside. Soon, we got word that all my tests were unremarkable. Except for one. A nurse with a tight onyx bun showed me a small, plastic wand. The precautionary pregnancy test. One line was dark pink (the control), the other a pink so faint I almost missed it. Impossible, I said, and insisted on a confirmatory blood test. It, too, was positive.

So at the moment I thought I was to die, I learned I was instead to give new life.

The doctor discharged me in a state of shock. David felt the same. Neither of us could grasp what had happened, or its implications. I sat up slowly, feeling like I had a hangover plus the flu, and stumbled twenty feet to the exit. David tried to help, but I felt clumsier with another person touching me. This was nothing like the last pregnancy. Nothing like the thyroiditis. Nothing like I had seen as a doctor.

Desperate for answers, I sat on a bench as we waited for my parents to come around in a taxi, and shuffled through my discharge papers. The diagnoses were vague ("dehydration, dizziness, pregnancy"). The screening labs were unhelpful ("within the reference range"). The discharge instructions were nonspecific ("Get immediate follow-up in America"). With nothing there to ground me, I withdrew into myself. It was the only thing I could do to keep from coming altogether undone.

My parents and Rosa arrived in a taxi van, and David and I piled in. It was dusk, and the solid gray canopy had turned to charcoal. All of us exhausted, the first ten minutes of the ride to my parents' house were silent. Then David spoke.

"Can you ask the driver to drop me off here?" he said, showing my parents an address on his phone.

"Where are you going?" I asked. He couldn't speak the language and didn't know his way around.

"There's a pick-up game organized by expats starting shortly."

"You're gonna play basketball *here, now*?" I said.

"I really need this game."

I said nothing. What could I have said? "I'm terrified of dying, oh, and by the way, I'm pregnant, so please don't leave me?" To have to ask for such a thing, to demand love, if that was even possible—I withdrew back into myself.

"I'll find my way back to the house," David said, as the van pulled up to the gymnasium.

And off he went.

At my parents' house, I tucked Rosa in for the night, then gathered my water bottle and some Tylenol. "Do you need anything else?" my mother asked. My hope for this trip had been for us to understand each other better, to show her I was fine on my own, and to come to a place of self-possession. But I couldn't even stand on my own two feet now, and my husband was off somewhere. At least I could try not to be a burden. "No, thanks," I said. "I'll try to get some rest."

I ignored my symptoms long enough to think. Putting things together, I concluded that my condition was a combination of dehydration from the hike, some strange food reaction, perhaps the mushrooms, and the early hormone shifts of pregnancy. Still in mental shock and feeling alone, I curled up under the covers, hoping to put this nightmare behind me.

At some point after the sky had turned from charcoal to black, the front door opened. My parents were watching a Chinese soap opera in the living room, and I could hear David talking to them. He entered our room with his face flushed, his T-shirt soaked in sweat. Quiet, I watched him strip off his clothes and socks and throw them in the corner. He didn't hop in the shower right away. He sat in his boxers on the edge of the bed near my feet, as though waiting to say something. As he started twirling his wedding band around his finger, I thought about the past two years, which now felt like a mountain of sacrifices—to restrain my frustrations, to be tender, to have sex despite how I was feeling inside—and couldn't force myself to reach out yet again. I was thinking about the inscription we had chosen for our wedding bands a mere four years earlier. Was it *Love* endures all things? Love *endures* all things? Or, Love endures *all things*? I didn't know. None of the versions rang true.

David finally broke the silence. "I really needed the—"

"I know."

"Do you need anything?"

As another wave of fatigue washed over me, I knew what I needed. "I need you to leave me alone."

Our scheduled departure was three days later. I hadn't recovered much and was worried about the thirteen-hour flight home. If I sat upright for more than a minute or two, my heart would race as though I was climbing a steep hill, leaving me dangling on the edge of passing out. At the airport, I needed a wheelchair to get to the gate. Rosa climbed onto my lap, holding her blanket and doll. I closed my eyes to filter out all the commotion, opening them when a stranger started scolding me to give the wheelchair to someone who really needed it. "I need it," I explained. You don't look sick, her eyes glared. A wall of eyes glared behind her.

But by some miracle, I made it onto the plane, and there was even room to lie down.

In the first twenty-four hours of being back in San Francisco, all three of us developed vomiting and diarrhea. I deemed it a gastroenteritis, probably a virus, probably caught on the plane (since my parents had no symptoms). We spent two days on the L-shaped couch, drinking ginger ale, nibbling on saltines, and sleeping on and off. Sometimes David and I talked about the news, sometimes the weather, sometimes work and other logistics, but not the trip, its events, or how we were feeling about any of it.

On the third day, I called my medical director to explain the gastroenteritis. I also broke the news to him of my surprise pregnancy, as I knew it might delay my recovery by a day or two. "I expect to be back at the clinic next week," I told him.

But I wasn't.

SEVEN

After the sudden disturbance in Beijing, my health would never be the same. I didn't understand it yet, that my autonomic nervous system—the branch of the nervous system that acts largely unconsciously and regulates vital functions like breathing, blood pressure, heart rate, and digestion, as well as influencing hormones and the immune system—had been thrown completely off, and as a result, my entire body was now under fire. Focused on a quick recovery, thinking I would soon get on with my life, I called my medical director every few days to tell him, "Sorry, just a few more days of rest."

Following the standard of care for any woman with a history of hypothyroidism who became pregnant, I started a low dose of levothyroxine, the synthetic thyroid hormone I had taken before. It wasn't a treatment dose; rather, a fraction of my original dose, simply to support the demands of pregnancy. With rest and fluids and time, the gastroenteritis passed. I assumed the profound fatigue and dizziness would pass, too. But I lay in bed for weeks, bound by what felt like a persistent flu and a panoply of what I called "accessory symptoms":

Vertigo, like the floors were sloping and the walls moving.

Brain fog, waxing and waning.

Internal tremors in the back and chest.

High-pitched ringing in the ears.

Lightheadedness, worse when sitting or standing.

Intermittent "undertows," suspending me on the verge of passing out.

Heart palpitations. Skipped beats, rapid thunder, irregular gallops.

Muscle aches, like I had run a marathon.

Frequent urination, especially at night.

Windedness, even at rest.

Stiffness in the fingers.

Numbness and tingling in the thighs.

Skin outbreaks, pimples and rashes.

Persistent nausea.

To move, I felt like a puppeteer pulling flimsy strings to get the life-sized doll moving, but there was hardly any energy to pull the strings. The only times I got out of bed were to use the bathroom or get some food. On a good day, I made it to the back deck to sit long enough to watch the wild parrots fly overhead. Sometimes I tried Dramamine, an over-the-counter remedy for motion sickness, but it made me too groggy. I stayed away from other medications, even ibuprofen, because of the pregnancy (my stomach couldn't have tolerated them anyhow). Sometimes I felt better after a bowl of broth. Eventually, I figured out that salty fluids helped the dizziness.

It was hard to manage while David was at work, especially with Rosa. I called on anyone that was available. David's parents rearranged their schedules to take Rosa more often. We increased Ayi's hours. Juan Carlos and other neighbors chipped in. David arranged for friends to drop in from time to time. But I couldn't tolerate anyone's presence. Not out of introversion, but due to the excruciating hypersensitivity to everything around me, ten times what it had been in the past. Visitors had to sit quietly, and even then, their breathing felt too strong, like they were sucking the residual energy out of me. Our bedroom became a dark cave.

On shorter work days, David would pop his head into the cave and ask in an expectant tone, "Did you have a better day?" I didn't like to say no. It seemed to disappoint him, and any tension between us would suck more energy out.

"Did Ben bring by some food?" he asked one evening.

"Couldn't eat it. Felt like throwing up. Asked him to leave. No social energy."

David's shoulders slumped. "What is it you want?"

I wanted to be alone. I didn't want to be alone.

On occasion, the symptoms would acutely worsen, and my heart rhythm would stampede across my chest as it had in Beijing, and the sensations in my body, which were already intolerable, would escalate. More than once, I cried out, "I can't take this anymore!"

"What is it you want?" David would ask again.

I couldn't say what I wanted because beyond the symptoms was something more paralyzing: the fear of death, knocking with every heart palpitation, pulling with each undertow, and taunting me with the continuous dizziness. Almost as bad as death was a state that felt like dying—the process of gradually ceasing to function, the *ehhh* sound between the two hard *d's* of the word *dead*. Sometimes the final *d* sounded like mercy to end the *ehhh*, but how could I really know? If I admitted this, it might put David, in whose eyes I could already see terror, into more of a doing mode. What if he told others and they prescribed antidepressants or psychotherapy? I wasn't depressed. I was miserable.

I wanted to die. I didn't want to die.

"I'm taking you to the emergency room," David would say.

"I don't want to go!"

He would take me anyhow, and the ER doctors would take my blood and urine samples and run their tests. The adrenaline-soaked environment sent electrical shocks through my body. The one grace would be the bolus of IV fluids, which would temporarily boost my blood pressure and help the dizziness. But when the tests came back normal, as they always did, the doctors would discharge me in NAD, or "no acute distress," and conclude, "This is just a difficult pregnancy."

"I know it's something more," I would plead. I had only one thing to go by—my subjective experience that my inner workings were all scrambled up. It didn't require a medical degree to know the difference between a shift in normal physiology, which was what pregnancy was, and a clear pathology. But the objective numbers, the numbers I once swore by, were betraying me. In the first month after the sudden disturbance, for acute episodes of feeling like I was drowning into myself, I was in and out of the ER three times.

As incapacitated as I was, I needed more answers. I took my heart palpitations and dizziness to a cardiologist. She noted my vital signs but said, without so much as an inflection in her voice, "I see this a lot." She wasn't concerned, she said, despite my erratic heart rate. To realize I had landed on the dark side of the biases that women, more often than men, were deemed exaggerators of their symptoms and were taken less seriously, caused anxiety to well up inside me. I knew I wasn't exaggerating.

She ran through a list of questions so fast that I, a trained internist, had a hard time following them. Over the next weeks, I underwent a series of tests, which picked up some irregular heart rhythms, but nothing that correlated with any of my symptoms. She offered a medication to control the arrhythmia by slowing my heart rate down, but dizziness and fatigue were common side effects. I respectfully declined.

The visits and tests made my symptoms more brittle. So I ensured at least a week of rest before seeing a neurologist for the weakness and tingling. The neurologist, like the ER doctors, attributed everything to a difficult pregnancy. "If your symptoms persist after you deliver the baby, come back and see us."

My next stop on the merry-go-round was to a psychiatrist. This was where all patients like me ended up sooner or later. I was surprised no one had referred me to one yet. Perhaps they were reluctant because I was a fellow doctor. Perhaps it was because I was pregnant. I was frightened I would discover that this was all in my head, that my emotions were creating these symptoms, but I still needed answers. During the thirty-minute evaluation, I lay on a couch as the psychiatrist asked her questions, scribbled on a notepad, then said something straight out of a comedy of errors: "I think it's your hormones. I recommend you see your endocrinologist."

Could I? The endocrinologist? The one who had put me through undue distress with the thyroid scan? There were others I could see, but he knew my case better than anyone else, and I was too tired to start fresh. With mixed feelings, I made an appointment.

Two years had passed since my last visit. The doctor's eyebrows looked bushier, and his voice had a new furry quality to it. His attire was the same, a pressed Oxford shirt buttoned all the way up, cinched with a bow tie. I was lying on my side on the exam table, curled up in a fetal position.

"Hello, Cynthia," he said, giving a formal nod.

"I really hope you can help me," I said, listlessly. "I'm in my first trimester of my second pregnancy, and I've been bed-bound for almost two months. I can hardly sit up. I'm exhausted—it's hard to describe how deep it is—and I have heart palpitations all the time. Do you think this could have anything to do with my thyroid?"

"Let's slow down for a moment. One symptom at a time." *Of course,* I thought. *But all my symptoms are related.* He tapped the keyboard with his index finger, one stroke at a time. "Let's see.... I believe your thyroiditis resolved."

"It did. And I'm taking a low-dose of levothyroxine for the pregnancy."

"Good." He turned the monitor to face me. "Your labs look great, even the ones from your most recent ER visit. Everything's within the reference range."

The reference range is a set of numbers that represents ninety-five percent of a sampled population, *n*, similar to a bell curve. I had always believed these tests to be diagnostic—definitive. But as I looked at the reference range from where I lay, the range looked wide. Very wide. And one of my hormone tests was on the far end of the curve.

"Could it be that the ideal level *for me* is a little different?" I was asking for an *n* of 1, not of thousands.

He looked puzzled, then somewhat offended.

I was desperate, so I tried to clarify, despite knowing what I was about to ask wasn't the standard of care. "Do you think I could adjust my levothyroxine dose and see if I feel better?"

"Your thyroid is fine."

He glanced at the clock, and I realized we were short on time. But I had one last concern to squeeze in. "What can I do this time around to lessen my chances of a thyroiditis flare-up postpartum?"

"Thyroiditis is genetic."

I understood the genetics, I said, then recalled some identical-twin studies determining that if one got thyroiditis, the other had a fifty to seventy percent chance of developing it. The "genetic" part, then, was a genetic predisposition, not a genetic predetermination, and the remainder was environmental.

"It's genetic," he affirmed.

Hearing his next words, I felt like I was lying in the Patient Lab of medical school, listening to rehearsed lines. "If any thyroid issues arise, come back and see us. Your primary care doctor can handle the rest."

Back at home, I collapsed on the bed. I didn't cry. Way beyond tears, I was in total defeat. How had this happened? Just a few months ago, I was a conqueror of thyroiditis, and now I was being passed around from specialist to specialist, neither *here* nor *there*, getting nowhere but dead-ends, which could only mean one thing:

I had become a difficult patient.

My life came to a standstill. David and I were mired in mundane logistics—Rosa, the house, the bills. Juan Carlos sometimes acted as an interpreter between David-ese and Cynthia-esc. But everything circled back to my health. My health this, my health that. I couldn't stand it, and yet it was the only thing we could talk about. For a few weeks, I tested out a higher dose of levothyroxine to see if it would help. It only aggravated the jitteriness and anxiety. To cope, I tried to detach from my body and focus on the present. If my mind were to delve anywhere, it was deeper.

David's strategy was to live as though nothing was different, fully in his body, pushing forward, the faster the better—because festive gatherings and new hobbies and planning ahead had the potential to push him past the hard stuff. He continued to invite friends over to watch political debates, discuss books on social change, or watch movies. All while I was in my cave.

He tried to help matters by taking a two-month sabbatical. Having gotten a generous offer to work in the solar industry of Silicon Valley,

David could take some time off between jobs. His salary would double, his benefits would increase. In the past year, he had become a rising star in his field, sitting on various boards of environmental organizations, consulting with government agencies, and advising local politicians. While I knew what a gifted mind he had for this work and how much he could impact the fight against climate change, the ease with which he moved through life was such a stark contrast to my state of being that it grated on me. I couldn't receive his gesture as a gift.

On the first day of his sabbatical, he introduced himself as House Hubby Extraordinaire. "I thought I'd do a grocery run today. Is there anything you'd like to request?"

"Could you lower your voice?" I whispered. It sounded like he was shouting.

"Why are we whispering?" he said, looking at Rosa, who had entered my cave. They shrugged their shoulders, giggled, and made fake whispering sounds.

"No noise, *please*," I said.

He put his index finger over his lips, signaling to Rosa to keep quiet. He handed me a piece of paper with a partial food list, to which I added several items.

"I'll get the groceries," he whispered. "You get some rest."

He made it sound so easy. The insomnia had continued to plague me intermittently over the past two years, and now, the exhaustion seemed to conversely rev up my systems—another result of the autonomic nervous system dysfunction I didn't yet know about. I was in "fight-or-flight," the stress state of the autonomic nervous system, which primes the body for acute survival: increased blood to the muscles and increased heart rate to prepare for flight, decreased blood to the gut and kidneys, which aren't deemed important in this survival state, and suppression of the immune system. In healthy physiology, once the acute stress is removed, the body shifts back into "rest-and-digest"—the state of long-term health as opposed to short-term survival. In rest-and-digest, digestion becomes active, the immune system works better, and overall health maintenance ensues. But in perpetual fight-or-flight, I was unable to rest or heal. I spent most of the morning staring at house-plants and following a gnat with my eyes.

Hours passed. When they returned, David entered, flooding the cave with the afternoon sun. "How was your day?" he said. "What did you do?" The questions highlighted my uselessness. "Did you get out to the deck?"

"No."

"Did you—?"

"No."

When Rosa came running in, he showed me some big plywood boxes. "Guess what these are." I shrugged my shoulders. He told me about a presentation by the San Francisco Beekeepers Association at the children's museum, how he had always wanted to learn beekeeping, and his sabbatical would be a great time to learn. Then he pulled out a beekeeper suit and a smoker, and started to assemble his hive kit. Rosa slipped her legs into the beekeeper suit, and he threw the mesh hat over her head, making her cackle. "A few weeks from now, I'll pick up some Italian honeybees, and at the end of the summer, we can harvest our first batch of honey."

Honey. End of summer. All the enthusiasm.

After they left, I closed my eyes, trying to escape mentally. Across the insides of my lids, the South African savanna played like a movie in Technicolor. One of the highlights of David's and my six-month travels was a leave-no-trace camping safari along the Umfolozi River. I could see the grasses, which were thick, brown, and waist-high. The spring water, the color of café au lait. Two guides holding their rifles. Mosquitoes buzzing, ticks bouncing. The yellow sun hanging in the horizon. The animal trails wove around riverbanks, rocky plateaus, and vast stretches of grassland. I could hear frogs croaking and lions grunting. I saw myself lying in a sleeping bag at night, staring at the flickering campfire, smoke evaporating into the black sky, a sky whose darkness was sprinkled with the glitter of the Milky Way. It was a different lifetime.

The next afternoon, my medical director called. I had been sending him email updates on a weekly basis, and I knew this call could only mean one thing: Could I return, and when, and if not, would I quit? My position was part-time and without benefits, so taking a medical leave meant quitting. With no diagnosis and no prognosis, I had no choice but to leave my position. Feeling the loss in my gut, I put away my white coat and scrubs, which were clean and folded. I took my pager and ID badge and put them in the closet, too. My pocket reference guides, my stethoscope, my reflex hammer…all into storage boxes. It felt as though I was leaving town for good. In a way, I was.

In the evening, David asked me, "Good talk with your supervisor?" He was sitting on the edge of the bed and snacking on popcorn.

"So…I had to take a medical leave." I couldn't say the word *quit*.

"You mean you quit?"

"I'll reapply when I'm ready to return."

"When will that be?"

"You think I have any clue?" I barked.

At the raising of my voice, David offered me some popcorn. It took everything I had not to knock the bowl out of his hands.

"We can make it on my income," David said, trying to offer something. "We'll be fine. We have a lot saved up. And hey, money is something we rarely fight about. You don't know how much I appreciate that you don't buy a lot of things. I love that you don't like to shop. I love that you're thrifty. I love—"

"That's not the point," I snapped.

"You've already accomplished so much."

"That's not the point, either!"

David had no way of winning this argument. On top of everything else, I was losing the identity that had been my ballast through all the past ups and downs. It was the one variable I could control—the variable that hadn't changed when Kurt died, or when I picked up and moved across the country, or when I got married, or even when I quit and traveled abroad, then returned. And this faithful variable gave me autonomy. When David and I had met, I was making twice his salary. Now I was fully dependent on him. This vulnerability made it impossible to receive his support as kindness. Nor could I receive as a kindness the privilege of having medical coverage through his job and the mercy of bypassing disability coverage, thereby being spared additional stigma, the hassles of paperwork, the stresses of having to weigh health against food or shelter or other basics, and the task of hunting down a doctor to fill out the paperwork in the first place. All these things I knew from the doctor side to be excruciatingly difficult. But in the moment, my patienthood was all-consuming.

As another bout of acute vertigo struck me—and worse, as the undertow threatened to pull me under—I saw that David had left the cave, defeated. I was on my own, clutching onto the bed frame, hoping to stabilize my inner workings by stabilizing my outer self. My limbs began tingling in an awful way—not like they were asleep, but like they were dissolving. A black hole seemed to appear on the ceiling, swirling like a whirlpool, and I wondered, terrified, if that was the *other* realm. Whatever it was, I felt it pulling, pulling.

It was there, in this darkest moment, that I felt a *pop-pop-pop*. After a brief pause, I felt the black hole pulling me in again. Then *pop-pop-pop* again, deep in my center. Little popcorn kernels were jumping to and fro, the somersaults and power kicks of the babe growing inside of me— the first perceived signs that, hidden under this mysterious illness was an explosion of life. Each pop seemed to say "I'm here!" They snapped me out of myself.

Other days, it was Rosa, tugging on my shirt or on my toes.

"Look!" she would say, and walk like a penguin.

"Look!" she would say, and dance a naked jig.

Other times, her tantrums expressed the raw urge to live. Her way or no way, daring anyone to contain her.

Once, she entered my room, carrying her favorite books in a tote bag: *Goodnight Moon. Good Night, Gorilla. Good Night, Good Knight.* I took them out, one by one, as she lay down on the floor, motionless.

"What are you doing?" I said.

"Shhhh," she said. (She had learned that from me.)

"What are you doing?" I repeated, in a whisper.

"I'm a poop," she whispered back, then lay her head down.

I cracked my first smile in months. For a few minutes, she did the near-impossible for a toddler—lie still—and pretended to be a piece of poop. After that, as we read through her books together, she held my bathrobe like a security blanket. By the end of the last *Good Night* book, she was asleep. I slipped a pillow under her head and wrapped my robe around her. "I'm sorry I haven't been able to play with you," I whispered, stroking her hair, "and haven't been able to put you to bed or to take you to the park." I rubbed her heels, and smelled her hair. Gazing upon her and feeling the babe in my center, I thought, *I have to get through this.* Two little beings depended upon me.

EIGHT

The surge of pregnancy hormones in the second trimester boosted my energy a notch. It was enough to resolve the feelings of dissolution and get me out of bed, sometimes even out of the house. I could manage basic housework, taking care of Rosa with Ayi's part-time help, and taking gentle walks for a block or two, all with the methodical movements of a precarious puppet. If a functionality score of 0 was bedbound and 10 was full health, I had been an 8–9 in my thyroiditis days, and now I lingered at 1–2. But the functionality score, however helpful to gauge overall changes, had its limits; it didn't capture how I actually *felt*. Like when I had the postpartum thyroiditis, I was almost fully functional—in terms of what David and others could measure—but on the inside, I felt on the verge of madness. Now, on a good day, I had an hour during which I could venture out for groceries or small errands. But the disequilibrium was constant and the fatigue threatened to worsen if I overexerted myself, so I never went far from home.

Ayi not only helped to clean, she became the only person I confided in with any regularity. She saw me in bed, and after a while, I grew comfortable with her seeing me unkempt. She helped me reorganize our flat, which our family was outgrowing. The baby would sleep in a bassinet in our room, and the fainting room, the size of a large closet, would become Rosa's room. As Ayi pulled out the newborn clothes from storage, she asked in an uncharacteristically direct manner, "What's wrong with you?"

"I don't know," I replied.

"But you're a doctor."

I was silent for a while, then changed the subject back to our flat.

David's sabbatical ended. He started his new job, with a long commute to Silicon Valley, so he left early and returned late. The long work days minimized the potential for friction between us, but at night, the friction remained. I longed for separateness, both for the hope of better sleep and for the relief from the pressures of sex.

I was married to a vibrant thirty-seven-year-old man. One who was supporting Rosa and me. One I had vowed to have and to hold in sickness and in health, and to love even when I didn't feel it. He had his basic drives. Sex was also his way to try to connect when we weren't connecting. For me, sex was something I wanted when I was *already* feeling connected, not something I used *in order to* connect. Besides, I couldn't even be in my body. Yet I felt I had to try. It was my effort to keep our relationship from becoming as brittle as my health. In some ways, trying to connect without words felt easier than speaking. But sex, once an uninhibited I-love-you and I-want-to-lose-myself-in-you, had become another checkbox on my growing list of to-dos, which were increasingly left undone.

During the second trimester, I underwent the standard obstetrics tests, ruling out anemia and gestational diabetes, and checking my thyroid levels, all within the reference range. At the prenatal ultrasound, we saw images of the baby, a large head and a shadow of limbs: ten fingers, ten toes, floating in a sea of black. I was relieved to know the baby's growth measurements, heartbeat, and movements were within normal parameters. When the baby started to suck his or her thumb, a rush of maternal love arose in me and I got choked up. I had been so focused on my illness, I hadn't recognized the important work my body *was* doing. As the test concluded, the tech asked if we wanted to know the baby's gender. David and I looked at each other. Who was this force of nature, I wondered, this being who had entered my life at the most trying of times?

It was a girl.

In his ongoing campaign to find *something* to support my healing, David brought in Juan Carlos, who offered what he was learning in acupuncture school. "In traditional Chinese medicine…" he would say, launching into something about too much dampness in the body. Or was it qi (pronounced "chee") stagnation? Or yin excess? The concepts made no sense to me because the organ systems in Chinese medicine didn't overlap with those in Western medicine. The body was understood in terms of energy, this mysterious qi whose flow mapped onto a network of "meridians."

"*Zu san li*," Juan Carlos said, his Mandarin sounding like a groaning Muppet. He was proposing an acupuncture point for general wellness.

Um, no thanks, I thought. This paradigm wasn't science-based. He might as well have been talking about the eyes of newts and roots of hemlock. Traditional medicine might work for him, but in my fragile, state I needed a lot more evidence.

When that failed, David flipped through his mental address book. "What about calling Pia?"

"Pia?" I said, my voice rising. Pia was a friend in her seventies whom we had met, along with her husband, Don, a few years earlier. A mutual friend of theirs and ours had been in a bad car accident, injuring her hip and requiring multiple surgeries. Pia stepped in to help. "She has a gift," our friend had explained. Pia could "see" things, and she had detected an infection in our friend's hip before the doctors did. "Are you serious?" I asked David now. "You think I should talk to Pia? She's a special person, but really, psychic stuff? I need sound medicine."

"Okay, okay," David said, backing off. "I wouldn't have suggested it if we weren't desperate. What about Yeshi?" Yeshi Neumann was a veteran midwife who had recently delivered our friends' baby.

"A midwife?" I said. "I need someone to help me with my health, not to deliver my baby. We've already got our obstetrician."

But thinking about the labor and delivery got me worried. I was two months away from my due date and couldn't imagine how I would have the energy to birth this baby. So after a few days of worrying about it, I asked for Yeshi's number.

On the day of her visit, the air was cool and foggy. I sat by the large bay windows watching for her, tracing droplets of mist along the glass. A Toyota Prius pulled into our driveway, and a woman with a silver bun stepped out. She wore an orange shawl, a white blouse, and blue jeans. Her dark eyes peered up at me, and I waved for her to come up. Before even introducing herself, she gave me a slow, deep embrace. Yeshi had an energy that felt at once novel and oddly familiar. Like I knew her without knowing her.

She took off her shoes and sat cross-legged on the living room floor. Over a cup of tea, she asked how I was, not in a clinical H&P way, but as if she were an old friend. I found myself opening up to her about my health, my pregnancy, and even my tensions with David. She listened without interruption. And when my concerns came to a natural end, she suggested we do a meditation together.

"I've never meditated before," I admitted, feeling ignorant in the presence of this wise woman. "How is it different than prayer?"

"It's more about clearing your mind and focusing on nothing."

"Clearing my mind? What would my mind *do*, then?"

She smiled, suggested I not overthink it, then asked me to lie down. Since clearing my mind felt difficult, she wanted to try guiding me through a meditation. Even before we started, I had the impression of being in a light hypnosis, completely open to her suggestions. My eyes closed, my body became heavy.

"Let your body sink into the cushions," she began. "Feel your body sinking… Let the couch support you… Below the couch is the floor, and below the floor are the support beams, and below the beams is the foundation, and below the foundation is the earth. Feel your body supported all the way down to the earth, which can hold everything, and let your body just fall completely into it."

After ten minutes, I opened my eyes, fully relaxed.

"Now in this state, Cynthia," she said, "I want you to feel your body and trust it. Trust that your body was designed to birth this baby."

As soon as I thought about my body, my relaxation vanished, replaced by anxiety. "What if I don't have the energy to deliver her?"

She asked me to describe the labor with Rosa.

I recounted how early in my labor, I spiked a fever; then the doctor gave me IV antibiotics to reduce the risk of a serious infection; but the antibiotics made me nauseated and I couldn't stop vomiting; then the nurses treated this with IV nausea medication; but the medication made me delirious; then I got an epidural; but the anesthesia stalled my labor.

This cycle of treating my symptoms, then treating the side effects of the treatments, continued until the last stage and left me depleted. Rosa's arrival had somehow erased all the traumatic memories, and recalling them now made me even more worried about how I would fare with the next one. I didn't know what Yeshi's role would be, but I already knew without a doubt that I wanted her in the delivery room.

"Do you remember when you hit your wall?" Yeshi asked. "I'm looking for the moment you thought, *I can't do this anymore, give me the epidural.*"

"Um, I guess when I was sitting by the toilet, vomiting, and the contractions were so strong and so close together that I wanted it all to go numb."

She responded with something that blew my mind. In her forty years of midwifery, she said, most often when a woman hit her wall, it wasn't from the pain itself. The contractions were, of course, very intense, but they came...*and they went.* The spaces between the contractions were often overlooked. They were precious moments of peace, whether they were several minutes or thirty seconds. If those moments weren't harnessed—if they filled up with anguish from the last contraction or worry for the next one—the pain could feel continuous. Then it would feel like ten or twenty or thirty hours of contractions, and no one could tolerate that.

Suddenly, I saw her point. It reminded me of the Japanese concept of *ma* I had learned about in college. *Ma*, which meant "gap" or "pause," is the negative space in buildings, like the openings under doorways and within fireplaces, or the spaces outlining the contents of a room. So if a space feels cluttered, it's not because of an excess of things, per se, but a deficiency of *ma*. *Ma* isn't an actual "thing." It's created by one's consciousness. This helped me understand the focus on nothingness in meditation, and its application to the labor process. My God, I thought, this concept could even apply to my marriage and health challenges.

When we said good-bye, she agreed to see me every other week. As my due date neared, or if I started having more activity in the belly, she would visit more often or check in by phone. My assignment was to practice focusing on the in-between spaces.

So I trained my eyes to see the negative spaces within the door frames. And played with optical illusions by Escher, switching back and forth between the two different perspectives. And stared at the non-forms between my outstretched fingers. I also practiced visualizations, seeing places in my mind's eye that evoked peace and warmth. Though I couldn't see it then, Yeshi was guiding me away from the hard, black outlines of life to looking anew for the colored textures within.

My belly grew larger.

The winter rains came.

Then the storms.

On a night when the gales were knocking out power lines and blowing palm fronds into the streets, I went into labor. My uterus contracted with amazing force, and this labor progressed much faster than the first. By the time we arrived at the hospital, I felt between my legs the urgency with which this force of nature wanted to enter the big world.

Yeshi met us there. Slipping off her raincoat, she directed David's hands to my lower back, and told him to apply counter-pressure.

"Don't be afraid of the pain," she said to me, "move *toward* it." I did what she said, and to my amazement, the pain lessened. Then she moved up to my ear and whispered, "All the mothers who came before you are sending their energy to you." A shiver flashed through me, giving me a burst of superhuman energy.

Over the next few hours, she encouraged me to visualize. Everything else had been a rehearsal, and this was the real performance. The stale hospital room transformed into a coral island in the South Pacific. During the rising contractions, I would ride them as a turtle riding the tremendous swells in the ocean. At the count of twenty, Yeshi would inform me that the crest had peaked, and as the swells began to wane, I would ride out the surf toward the shore. During the in-between spaces, I would imagine myself still a turtle, sunning myself on the warm, golden sands of a beach that stretched out forever.

I didn't know how I did it. I wasn't even positive it had happened. But when I emerged from the space between form and non-form, there she was—my babe, still moist, snuggled against my chest.

NINE

2008

We named her Sonia. Her skin was olive, her hair espresso, and her eyes gray. I fell into a love affair with her, as I had with Rosa, and for the first few weeks, I wouldn't let her leave my side. Her energy was soft yet intense. She often gazed into my eyes for several minutes at a stretch without a single cry or fidget. I felt attuned to her silence, and she to mine, as though she knew silence was what I needed. I was riding on a high, partly from the hormones, partly from the wonder of the birthing process. *I did that?* I kept thinking. *My body actually did that, and without pain medication?* I was also producing breastmilk, and plenty of it. All of this felt like a huge mystery, given how deficient my body was.

Yeshi paid us a few postpartum visits, checking on Sonia and me. Once, when I lamented all that I couldn't do for my children, she reminded me to see the in-between spaces. "You're home right now. Take this as a gift. If you're emotionally present for them, that's what they'll remember." So I nursed my baby and held her close.

During the pregnancy, I had been holding on to fragments of hope that my inner workings would restore themselves after the birth. But with each passing day that my symptoms persisted, that hope dwindled. In fact, my health declined. My nervous system became so easily triggered that I had to avoid anything that might cause stress or excitement, lest it aggravate my fatigue and dizziness, which would then trigger anxiety, which would then worsen my fatigue and dizziness. So I stopped driving on anything other than small roads, stopped playing the radio, stopped watching action movies, and stopped reading intense novels or the news. More than shielding myself from the world, though, I was trying to shield myself from me.

My already small world grew smaller.

I asked my parents to come for the Chinese tradition of *zuo yue zi* ("sitting the month"), a thirty-day confinement period for postpartum recovery. *Zuo yue zi* rules can vary, from the new mother being forbidden to wash her hair or brush her teeth, to not being allowed to eat cold foods or watch television. Two things, however, are generally agreed upon: (1) no visitors except close family and friends, and (2) no sex. I took this as permission to relax from marital pressures. But these rules further widened the distance between David and me.

I did whatever my mother prescribed, even when I didn't understand the rationale. "Don't eat bananas on an empty stomach," she would say, mixing Mandarin and English, and "Don't expose your ankles to cold air," and "Don't eat spicy foods." In her presence, I resorted to doing as I was told, trying somehow to right all the times I had missed the mark as a child. The best part was the homemade soups and congees made with oxtail or fish heads or salty rice, which my mother rotated day to day. Despite having no appetite, I finished everything because an empty bowl was a token of love. Privately, I yearned for her to stop the busyness and sit with me. She didn't need to say anything.

I never really let my parents know how awful I was feeling. I didn't know how. For the Chinese, burdens are never put on others. I knew my parents carried their own unspoken burdens—pains I would never know. And while they knew about my postpartum thyroiditis and had been there for the sudden disturbance in Beijing, they didn't know much about what was happening now, and they didn't ask. I knew they could see my diminished state, and figured they would ask if they really wanted to know.

On the days I couldn't get out of bed, my mother checked in with my health, albeit indirectly.

"Have you been praying?" she said, one afternoon.

"No," I confessed. I hadn't prayed since college, when I had left my parents' church and declared myself agnostic.

"You need to pray more," she said. "Ask God to heal you."

My shoulders tensed. A discussion about God was the last thing I wanted right now. In an effort to connect with her, though, I tried. "I don't really understand how faith works, Mom. How do I make myself believe in a Being or a Spirit who allows so much suffering?"

She walked around the room, flipping through our mail on the desk, looking at the stamps. "Faith is believing in something you can't see," she said, referencing an idea I had heard growing up, one I had even jotted down in my journal. I didn't fully understand it then, and I didn't know what to do with it now. She asked if she could tear off some stamps for her collection. I said sure. She nodded, affirming that she had said what she wanted to say.

On the day of fish ball soup, thirty days after they had arrived, my parents returned to Beijing. Their visit was a real gift to us. I thanked them. They said they would continue to pray for me, and I knew they would. I walked them to the front door, saw them off, then decided to take my first walk outside the house in a month. I felt stiff and unsteady with each step, conveniently using Sonia's stroller as a walker.

"One day at a time," David yelled from the front steps.

One step at a time, I thought.

A few months later, at month four, round two of the postpartum thyroiditis flared up. Round two was just like round one—a hyper- then hypo- roller-coaster. Except this time, my numbers didn't normalize. By diagnostic criteria, this meant the postpartum thyroiditis had evolved into chronic hypothyroidism or "Hashimoto's"—more a name change than a change in underlying pathology. The treatment for Hashimoto's, as I understood it then, was simply to take thyroid replacement for the rest of my life; in all likelihood, my dose requirements would increase over time. Taking the medication kept my levels within the reference range, but given my panoply of symptoms going into it, not surprisingly, nothing except my numbers improved on the medication.

My new normal was hypothyroidism, and *then some.*

Then some meant some kind of syndrome. Syndromes are names for clusters of symptoms where the effects are widespread and the causes poorly understood. That is, there isn't one organ that can be identified as the culprit, and there are no catchy mnemonics to explain the cause. To have any chance at treatment, I needed a diagnosis. The words of my mentor Dr. Eisenberg came to mind: "A good H&P will tell you 90 percent of what you need to know." Could I take my own history and physical and try to deduce what I had? Then, could I muster the mental energy to do some research on the computer?

One morning, after having a big sandwich and a glass of salty water, I grabbed my home monitors and doctor's tools and stood naked in the bathroom. Temperature, 97.1 degrees Fahrenheit. *Below average.* Resting heart rate, 82. *Fast.* Blood pressure, 90/62. *Normal, but might be too low if I'm dizzy.* The rest of my exam was mostly unremarkable. But if I looked at my appearance, I looked like someone with a long-standing flu—dusky skin, sunken eyes, dry lips, an inability to stand fully upright. I knew from my previous labs that I wasn't anemic and, beyond generalized fatigue and dehydration, I didn't know what these physical signs meant.

After five minutes or so, I felt my heart rate climbing. I rechecked my vital signs—heart rate 122 while merely standing. Blood pressure, unchanged. A marked rise in heart rate while standing indicated autonomic dysfunction, or the dysregulation of the branch of the nervous system that controls largely unconscious and vital functions, the inner workings that had snapped during the sudden disturbance in Beijing. This finding was the key to narrowing down my potential diagnoses.

I got dressed and researched online, putting my cursory H&P together. My assessment concluded with two names, which I jotted in my journal:

Chronic fatigue syndrome

Dysautonomia

The satisfaction that comes with a diagnosis was blatantly absent. Chronic fatigue syndrome is a lump term for someone with debilitating fatigue and immune and neurological dysfunction, whose symptoms worsen with minimal to moderate exertion. Dysautonomia is simply a fancy term for autonomic dysfunction, which means the signals are crossed and the fight-or-flight stress state dominates over the rest-and-digest healing state. Basically, the syndromes summed up my symptoms without telling me anything more.

The therapies usually entailed a cocktail of antidepressants, anti-inflammatories, psychotherapy, and, in prolonged cases, immune-suppressing drugs. I had no interest in any of the potential side effects of these treatments. I wasn't even interested in suppressing my symptoms. I wanted to know what the hell was actually going on, and how to heal!

While I couldn't find much in the way of statistics for dysautonomia, in chronic fatigue syndrome, less than half improved, and only about five percent made a full recovery. Worried these statistics could psychologically hinder any chances for recovery, I opted not to identify with the syndromes at all, except for research purposes. When people asked what was wrong with me, my answer was a simple "hypothyroidism," or "Hashimoto's."

I tried to remember my patients with some version of this. Like the one who had asked about "chronic mono," and countless others who had complained of ongoing fatigue or dizziness. I had referred them to various specialists, who ran numerous tests, often without much conclusion. Sometimes the doctors cast wider nets, but without knowing what they were fishing for, then having to confront the problem of "incidentalomas"—ambiguous findings like a spot on the lung or a mass on the adrenal glands. What then? More testing, more invasive procedures, more expense, more trauma. In the end, most patients had more questions than answers. So logically, I had assumed my patients' conditions weren't real. The only explanation seemed to be an emotional disorder.

Sitting with my self-diagnosis, I knew I didn't have the energy or the stability to handle such a workup. Even if I did, I would have run the other way. Hospitals and clinics as a whole, which had once been my home, a place that had defined me, now felt like settings in a dystopian novel. I holed up in the corner of my room for over an hour. Since I saw the perspective of both doctors and patients in these situations, I wasn't angry, but lost.

When Rosa came trotting in, I snapped out of my trance and looked down at my journal, still open in my lap.

"Whatcha doin', Mama?"

"I don't know," I said. "I don't know anything anymore."

I jotted down the next idea that came to my mind:

The paradigm works. Until it doesn't.

TEN

Accepting that the foundation of my life was crumbling was hard. Accepting my condition as a longer-term reality was harder. Changing Sonia's diapers, soothing Rosa's tantrums, doing the dishes, and engaging in other activities helped me stay relevant, useful. But as soon as I plopped onto the couch in between the busyness, my existential reality haunted me. David continued operating from his life-is-good stance, looking ahead to the chapter when things would return to normal.

"Don't you wanna know what's going on in the world?" he asked from behind *The New York Times* at breakfast one day.

"It's not that I don't care, it's that I can't handle it!" I bemoaned.

"Is there anything that *doesn't* make your symptoms worse?" he said.

Interpreting this as "Don't be so sensitive," I wanted to come up with something I could tolerate. National Public Radio? No. James Bond movies? No. Romantic comedies? Maybe. Reese Witherspoon? Yes.

David laughed.

"Maybe Woody Allen?" I knew I sounded ridiculous, but I wasn't just being high-maintenance. Hey, I wanted to shout, remember me, the woman who traveled the globe for six months with five shirts, two pairs of pants, a skirt, and five pairs of underwear; the one who ate whatever the locals ate and slept wherever she could find a bed, including cots under hole-ridden mosquito nets in malaria country? That's still me. But expecting him to believe my current experience—something he hadn't seen or experienced himself—was a case of that elusive thing called faith. I needed him to have faith. In me.

One night, I tried a Woody Allen classic, *Annie Hall*, halfway through which my vertigo kicked up. I looked over to find David surfing the Internet on his phone.

"Why are we even watching this?" I asked, frustrated.

"I don't know," he said, seemingly unaware of my efforts. "How 'bout something livelier, if you know what I mean?" He walked toward the bedroom.

I followed him and offered a compromise, which took all my composure. "How 'bout we snuggle instead? Like spooning, you know… naked, like we used to." I started to undress.

"You don't understand…for guys, that's basically impossible." In his boxer shorts, he headed out of the bedroom.

"If I don't want to have sex, you're moving to the living room?"

"It's hard for me to sleep next to you if I can't be relaxed."

There seemed to be no middle road.

The other major challenge was David's fast-paced life, which was getting faster. He wasn't a rising star in his field anymore; he was a full-fledged champion. When he wasn't at the office, he was traveling around the country and abroad, spearheading renewable energy policies wherever he went. A two-million-dollar grant here, a major policy breakthrough there. I couldn't keep up with his good news—enthusiasm fatigue, I called it. I hadn't known such a thing was possible, but there it was. The enthusiasm fatigue didn't generate friction between us unless it involved gatherings in our home. In addition to social gatherings, David was now hosting fund-raisers for grassroots groups, and dinner parties for dignitaries. I would always assess what my nerves could handle, and try to say yes to things that would push me beyond that. But he only seemed to see the no's. Whatever I offered never felt like enough.

This was a conversation we recycled I don't know how many times:

"I've already dialed my social life way down," he would say.

"You don't understand," I would say. "I'm barely holding on."

"I'm barely holding on, too," David would interject.

"What are you talking about?!"

He could never articulate it, except by saying, "I really need this."

I couldn't see it then, but for David, these experiences were more than just self-serving or frivolous. He was trying to keep our family and himself from sinking. And gathering people for a good, concrete cause gave him hope, nourished his soul, and grounded him. It was about staying alive in a different sense.

After a dinner party one night, he asked me, "How was that for you?"

"I'm tired!" I sounded like a parrot, one that only complained. "Please don't ask me anymore!"

"I told you before," he said, bringing the temperature down, "you don't have to lift a finger. You can rest all night in bed."

"But this is *our* home," I groaned, bringing the temperature right back up. "They're *my* guests, too. So if they're here, I wanna be partners in this. I want the house to be clean and the food to be good. And I need people, too. I want to engage with them as much as I can. I mean, who wants to spend all night in bed?"

David looked at me with an expression of *What the hell?*, and I realized I was contradicting myself. I didn't want people around, I wanted them around. I wanted to rest, I didn't want to rest.

"But then you blame me for making you tired."

"Because you do!" I could feel inflammation mounting in my shoulders and thighs. After a few moments to settle myself, I said, "I want a new solution, instead of repeating the same thing over and over again. I think we need a marriage counselor."

He shook his head. "I'm allergic to therapy of any kind, remember?" This was a reference to his parents putting him in therapy when he was in high school. He swore to steer clear of it from there on out.

"I know you had a bad experience before, but that was a long time ago. Besides, it's not like we're making a lot of progress on our own. We need to see one...or else."

"Or else what?" David said, with a rare sternness.

I didn't dare continue, lest I say something I would regret. So I grabbed a pillow and a blanket, and slept in the living room.

A month later, another rerun. We were cleaning up the garage after the inaugural honey harvest from the hives—fifteen or so friends, three different stations of equipment, topped off with a batch of honey lemonade. I had enjoyed seeing our friends and learning how to harvest the honey. But I anticipated feeling worse for the next few days, and resented David, as I saw it, for setting me up to fail.

"This is bad for my health," I said. There were studies that linked marital stress to inflammation and chronic diseases. Stressful marriages perpetuated partners' stresses, driving up stress hormones and suppressing the immune system, and I told David so.

He stopped scraping honeycombs off the floor. "Wait, are you saying I'm causing your health problems?"

"*Contributing* to them," I said, ignoring the dizziness that was kicking up.

"I feel like you're deliberately trying to extinguish my light."

"Wow," I said, offended. I was talking about *my* stress, but he had turned it into his. "If things are so bad for you...if I can't be social enough or sexual enough or anything enough for you...I mean, if I can't pull my own weight financially...if all we do is bring each other down, if you won't see a marriage counselor...if this just fucking sucks, why are we together?"

He sat down. "You think we should separate?"

For several minutes, I said nothing. Did I truly want to leave him? Or did I want him to see my pain? Or was I wanting to punish him, to even things out? I didn't know, and I couldn't sort through it because all the joints and muscles in my body hurt, and all I could feel was how much stress he brought to my life. Eventually, I said, "Yes. You and me together—it's making my health suffer." I felt clear about it until the words came out of my mouth. If David actually left, *then what?* Figuring out how to manage life alone, to support myself and the girls—or worse yet, knowing the girls might do better living with their healthy father...

"Please, at least look at me." His voice softened. "If you want me to leave, I'll leave."

There was a long silence.

"But I don't want you to worry," he added, his voice still soft.

I turned to face him. "About what?"

"Look, this is hell for both of us. But the last thing you need to worry about is money. I'll support you until you're able to work again."

His comment was like cold water on my face, an act of shocking compassion that reopened my eyes, long blinded by pain and anxiety, and suddenly, I could see his authenticity, decency, and love. Feeling ashamed and self-absorbed, I took a few steps toward him. Then in the garage window, through dust and cobwebs, I caught the creepy outlines of my reflection. The Gorgon!

And that's when another truth hit me like cold water: It was *me* I wanted to leave. Not him—*me*. It was my illness I wanted to leave. But my illness and I had become fused.

David held me for what felt like ten minutes. Then went upstairs and crashed into a deep sleep.

I cried soundlessly all night.

For weeks, I felt haunted by a shadow. What it was, my conscious mind couldn't quite perceive, but the dark energy was familiar, as if from a past life. It seemed to follow me throughout my days, and grew especially large when the flu-like malaise pinned me down.

One day, while resting in the bedroom, I eavesdropped on David, who was on a call about a big vote coming up in the state legislature. The world of politics had always been foreign to me, and I listened with awe and envy to the sophistication of his strategic mind. After he hung up, he made another call, instantly switching modes to plan a camping trip with a friend. This other David started talking about finding a site by a fresh lake so he could teach Rosa to fish. Then he entered the bedroom, changed into his basketball clothes, and said he was stepping out for a game.

I gasped. "Number Two." The shadow from a past life was coming into full light.

"What'd you say?" He grabbed his basketball shoes from the closet.

"Nothing. I was just talking to myself."

"Did you say 'number two'?"

I nodded reluctantly. Dealing with this illness, losing my identities and my voice…the world overwhelming me, closing me in, inch by inch...and watching how easily David moved through life, like he was dancing. This was how I had felt as a little girl—overly sensitive, invisible, powerless. All my health challenges were magnified by these formative stresses. It wasn't about competing with David, per se; it was about being lost as to who I was, and the current Number One further obscuring me.

I tried to explain, but he dashed off, saying, "Don't be ridiculous, second to who?"

Second to Superman, I thought. A superhero who comes from a superfamily, in a city of superheroes doing super things to save the world—that's who.

Later, I combed through a box of old photos, staring at the little girl in the home-sewn plaid dress, whose chin was tilted downward, eyes upward, thinking others couldn't see her if she couldn't see them. Then, at eleven or twelve, she sported winged bangs and her one and only Izod shirt, trying to play tough even if she wasn't inside, smiling with a full set of teeth, shoulders taller. This was around the time I had decided I hated being weak, and was done with it. I didn't know the concept of the "orchid child" yet, or the health risks of being sensitive; that these sensitivities could lead to exaggerated stress responses, which could lead to increased risks for chronic health conditions, including autoimmunity. All I had known was that I had a simple choice—continue more of the same, or find a new way—and had chosen the latter, holding in mind a singular question: How to build a thicker skin?

And now here I was, twenty-five years later, facing another critical choice: continue with more of the same and risk losing my beloveds, or find a new way. After the decisive fight with David, I knew this life was something I wanted to guard. The illness had taken so much already. I was determined not to let it take my beloveds, too.

I didn't know what I didn't know (a universe of wisdom). I also didn't know that this journey would take as long as it did (the better part of a decade, and counting). So it was with a sincere but naive resolve that I made the choice to find a new way.

My singular question this time: How to get off the couch?

Part Two

I hadn't a clue how to begin. It's not like I could finagle my way out of this dilemma by just toughening up, as I had when I was young. That hadn't worked anyhow. The thicker skin I had spent so much time building up had grown perilously thin. My greatest challenge was figuring out what my first step would be—then finding the motivation to take it. Not just because every action took three times as long to execute, but because lying down was one of the only activities I longed for. The couch had become my reward. I depended on its comfort after chores, childcare, and any kind of exertion. So I gave myself three months to enjoy it a little longer, procrastinating on my How to Get Off the Couch assignment.

Finally, come the winter holidays, I grew restless with myself, eager for change. The timing was fortuitous, because David was taking Rosa on their long-awaited camping trip, the first of many father-daughter trips to come. It would be infinitely easier to think without Superman around. And with Rosa three and a half, her world expanding at top speed, it was getting increasingly hard to keep up with her, too. Sonia, one now and weaned off nursing, would be easy to care for solo. As David and Rosa packed the car full of gear and waved good-bye, I exhaled, *Ahhh.* Now I could set my own pace; I could just *be.*

For two days, I did little besides watch Sonia totter around. We ate leftovers and frozen foods. No one came to the house. I let the chores pile up. Come Sunday morning, the last day of the camping trip, Sonia was still tottering—it felt as though she had never stopped—and I watched her from the couch, exploring the living room.

"Da!" she grunted, pointing to the blue tang in the saltwater tank.

"Fish," I said.

A few seconds later, "Da!" Her little finger pointed toward the toy basket.

"Doll."

"Da!" in the direction of the bookshelf.

War and Peace. Can you say, Lee-o Toll-stoy? Lee-ovv Nee-ko-lai-uh-veech Toll-stoy?"

Sonia gave me a blank stare, scooted in the opposite direction, and zigzagged across the living room. I had watched her on her feet for weeks now, but this time it was different. Now I really *saw* her. The astonishment at her own mobility, the tantalizing world beyond her reach, her eyes twinkling, her questions exciting her into a rage.

Once, I had that rage, too. It was just as I was embarking on the path to doctorhood. Somewhere during my training, the sense of discovery vanished, replaced first by a focus on survival—simply trying to survive the demands of medical boot camp—then a sense of mastery—I was saving patients, and to those I couldn't save, I provided drugs to ease their passage. I knew the drills and the protocols pat. Then came the loss of Kurt, leaving me numb. And now the illness, along with the challenges of parenting and marriage. I could come up with a laundry list of reasons why I had lost my quest for discovery. But they were excuses, not solutions. I had to follow Sonia's lead. It seemed I was less here for the girls' benefit than they were here for mine.

I pulled *War and Peace* off the shelf, searching for my lost learner self. Not there.

Sonia's *Da!* bellowed in the background as I raked the filing cabinet for my learner self, flipping through papers from college. Not there either.

When I came to the H&Ps I had written up for Dr. Eisenberg, the thickness of the stacks stunned me. I weighed them on my hand, as he used to. I read through them, line by handwritten line, the History of Present Illness alone taking up one page, front and back; the stories of war veterans I had interviewed and examined at the VA hospital, the words and tone reading as though written by someone else. *This was my learner self.* This was before I knew anything about drugs or fancy treatments. I had simply been trying to understand their stories.

Now, perhaps I had been making things too complicated by naming my conditions and figuring out what drugs would help.

I had to return to the basics.

To harness Sonia's *Da!*, I searched the kitchen for navel oranges. Instead, I grabbed what was available, a Meyer lemon, then found the sewing kit and made a simple interrupted stitch, the only suturing technique I could recall. Then I rummaged through the closet for my stethoscope. Since Sonia refused to sit still for even a second, I listened to my own heart. *Lub.* S1, the first heart sound, a low-pitched thump, the contractile phase when the heart pumps blood to the rest of the body. *Dub.* S2, the second heart sound, a higher-pitched snap, the opening of the chamber, when the heart relaxes and fills its empty chambers. *Lub-dub, lub-dub.* There was still lifeblood in me. A lot of it.

When the malaise kicked up, I put Sonia down for a nap and took a bath. It helped a bit, so I toweled off, and scanned my shelves for a book on the fundamentals. The *Pathologic Basis of Disease.* Of course! This was a 1,300-page textbook on the hows and whys of disease development. My very first purchase, it was dog-eared, highlighted, and still smelled like the medical school library.

I perused the first few chapters, following my old highlights and notations. Cell injury. Cell adaptation. Inflammation. Repair. In these chapters, I learned—or relearned—that diseases begin as subtle imbalances and low-grade inflammation for several years, sometimes decades, before a diagnosis can be made. That is, the "*here* you're well, *there* you're not" model wasn't true. There was no distinct line between health and disease. The state of health was *here* ⟷ *there*, a zipper-type continuum that moved in dynamic fashion between *here* (when cells got repaired) and *there* (when cells got injured). So I had to unlearn the idea that diseases and chronic conditions were determined by a fixed number or a positive test result, or fulfilling specific criteria.

This was a huge revelation.

Since the initial thyroiditis, my body had felt inflamed. But to my doctor's mind, indoctrinated by the *here/there* dogma, inflammation didn't qualify as a treatable disease. While acute inflammation was a protective response, chronic inflammation could be destructive. Inflammation in my balance centers could cause the dizziness. Inflammation of sensory nerves could cause the hypersensitivities.

Inflammation in the muscles could cause the aches and fatigue. This continuum meant that the opposite of disease—health—could be attained through a reversal of the zipper *here*-ward (toward repair). This was something I could control the pace of. Something my body might tolerate. And something that would move toward healing, as opposed to symptom management.

With that, I returned to the trusted scientific method. *Ask a question. Gather background research. Construct a hypothesis. Conduct an experiment. Analyze the data. Draw conclusions.*

Okay, I thought. *Ask a question.*

I already had one: How to get off the couch?

Next, *Gather background research.*

This much I knew: I have autoimmunity, widespread inflammation, and dysfunction of the nervous system.

Construct a hypothesis.

If I focus on righting my imbalances and inflammation, I can beat the odds and heal.

Conduct an experiment.

I'm my own doctor, I'm my own case study. An *n* of 1. Life *is* the experiment.

As I reflected on this paradigm shift, I knew my challenge was formidable: to sort through studies of reductionist science, which provided the necessary black-and-white information, and somehow apply them to the human experience, which was gray, gray, and more shades of gray. All that, on top of a foggy, slowed brain.

By the time the dynamic duo returned from their trip with fishing stories and woody treasures from the lakeshore, I was jotting my thoughts into my journal, reclaiming another tool that had been useful in the past—a list. This list, though, wasn't a handy tool for memorizing factoids. These were rules to live by. This experiment was going to be one part science, one part art, and one part faith. And now I had my first step.

How to Get Off the Couch

1. Ask new questions.

David and I were stuck in a zipper-type continuum, too. On one side was intimacy, on the other, autonomy; yet autonomy was also a precondition for healthy intimacy, so this got me confused about where to start. I knew that David's work demanded a lot of energy. And at home, since the children came first, we didn't have much energy left over to ask new questions in our marriage. I told myself I would settle for short-term coping skills instead of longer-term healing, and the first step was to reduce my heated outbursts. To really try, even if it meant detachment. I replaced the heat with a cool politeness, and I tried to harness Sonia's *Da!*, the new learner's mind, and apply it to David. I decided to steer us toward the theoretical and away from the personal.

So one Saturday, I explained the scientific method to him, along with how I was plotting my next steps. I worried he might think it too cerebral, but he nodded, said he liked the method, and that he was starting an experiment of his own. "Water from the standard faucet flows at two gallons per minute," he said, "but these new faucets have flow rates of half a gallon per minute." He had ordered some newer faucets to upgrade ours and was eager to see how much water we saved. Then he moved on to shower heads. Then energy-efficient lightbulbs. His rant faded into *wah-wah-wah-wah,* as he lost me in the numbers. The important thing was, we were awakening the art of discovery about issues we cared about. And as a result, we fought less.

In the arena of family life, I couldn't as easily escape the Number Two mindset. With Rosa an active toddler, David was taking her out more and more, to football games, political fund-raisers, and sometimes to his breakfast meetings. He also treated her to the things he loved, like Mitchell's ice cream. Since Newton's Third Law dictated that every action had an equal and opposite reaction, I felt I had to balance David's fun and sweets with sensible habits. My overcooked broccoli couldn't compare to his Rocky Road. My quiet play couldn't compare to his rowdy 49ers' fans. I feared that I couldn't compare to David in the girls' eyes.

At night, I would crawl into my shoebox—that's what my side of the bed started to feel like. We had one of those long body pillows that used to move from my side to David's side—whoever wanted it that night—but it now divided us. My side felt airless, cut off from all erotic experiences. A shoebox felt apt, since all dead things seemed to belong there. For our marriage's sake, I would try to crawl out of the shoebox and recall what raw pleasure felt like. But because I was trying to avoid seeing, hearing, tasting, or touching anything that might trigger my nervous system, I could only manage being half-in, half-out, and would lie there, stiff.

"Try to relax," David would say. I would try. Hard. But if I changed positions too quickly, I would become dizzier. Then I would worry about the palpitations, and they would indeed come—*thumpety-skip...thumpety-skip*—and I would have to breathe through them. Afterward, David would say, "How was that for you?" As I slept in the usual starts and stops, the long night would reveal to me the state of my soul—that if I longed for intimacy, I feared it more. Loving risked losing. So I was comfortable in the shoebox, because beyond the point of airlessness was an absolute safety. Dead things couldn't die again. No one could hurt me in there.

TWELVE

I knew my How to Get Off the Couch experiment had to start with improving my sleep. Otherwise I wouldn't have the energy to take any further steps. When Sonia was nursing, I had been resigning myself to poor sleep; but she was weaned now. My sleep had been poor even before health troubles and motherhood. Sleep deprivation was the norm, even commended, during medical training. In residency, we were, ironically, taught the importance of sleep with regard to our patients. Yet between monitors beeping, nightshift nurses dispensing medications or inserting IVs, and phlebotomists drawing blood at five a.m. so doctors could have results back by morning rounds, patients were lucky to get a couple hours of uninterrupted sleep. Doctors and patients alike were prone to lower energy, moodiness, and foggy memory. Not to mention the risk for conditions like cardiovascular disease, obesity, and the onset of autoimmune diseases.

Reunited with pathology basics, I plopped on the couch, researching online for why autoimmunity was linked to sleep troubles. There was a newly discovered system in the brain called "the glymphatics." This network of channels expands fourfold during the deepest stages of sleep. Like a crew of car washers, they flood the brain with fluid and remove the grime from the day's activities. In addition to the washers, a repair crew also enters during sleep, fixing areas damaged by aging, infections, and toxic chemicals. According to a lost-sleep calculator I found, at four hours of sleep per night, I was losing an average of eighty-four days' worth a year. Over a lifetime, this translated to enough lost sleep to watch 762 baseball games! Since I wasn't getting my nightly cleanse and repair, damage was likely building up. From there, inflammation could ensue.

And there was more. In patients with chronic fatigue, inflammation often builds up in the limbic system, the part of the brain that stores survival instincts, emotions, and memories. Inflammation in the limbic system can result in heightened anxiety and PTSD-type responses. And heightened anxiety can generate more inflammation in the brain. People stuck in this vicious cycle often feel their worlds getting smaller and smaller.

Bingo. This was me. My body didn't discriminate between emotional and physical stress after all—they were coals in the fire of inflammation either way. Inflammation didn't just make me feel achy and old, it also made me anxious and sleepless. The poorer my sleep, the greater the inflammation, and the greater the inflammation, the poorer my sleep. So it wasn't that these symptoms were in my imagination.

"Earth to Cynthia," David called.

I glanced up to see Sonia sitting on his shoulders. "Oh, sorry, I was reading up on sleep physiology."

"I thought I'd take the girls down to the park. You up for it?"

"I've got a lot more research to do."

"Come on," David urged. "The sunshine will get your cycles regular again."

While they romped in the playground, I sat on the bench where I used to sit when Rosa was a baby. The dogs were still running around on the hill, the sun was still shining over the cityscape, and the ice cream cart was still jingling its bells. The world was running like clockwork. David's off-the-cuff comment was actually a brilliant insight—it was more than just sleep. I had to get my whole internal cycle regular again.

As I thought about it, my insomnia had no real pattern. Sometimes I couldn't fall asleep, and stayed awake all night. Sometimes I fell asleep but woke after three or four hours, unable to fall back asleep. Sometimes I slept all night, but still felt groggy the next day. Whatever the trouble,

I was exhausted when I should have been awake and awake when I should have been sleeping. Even before my health troubles, my circadian rhythm had been off. Back in residency, after my thirty-six hour shifts, I would be tired but wired.

The circadian rhythm is an inner clock that follows the twenty-four hours in a day. The master clock sits in the master hormone gland in the middle of the brain, where it regulates the sleep-wake cycle and governs the clocks for the entire body. Each internal organ has its own clock, too, which is somehow coordinated by and with the master clock, so different functions turn on at different times of day. Next to the master hormone gland is a pine cone–shaped gland that makes melatonin, the hormone that induces sleep. The pine cone and the master gland talk to each other, synchronizing their roles to maximize a good night's rest.

When I learned that a disrupted circadian rhythm could cause inflammation, I got serious about regulating my days and nights. Since the circadian rhythm is sensitive to light-dark signals and artificial lighting confuses the brain, I reinstated what my father used to drill into us—*Early to rise, Early to bed*—even on weekends and holidays. I made a point of rising with the sun, avoiding napping in the afternoons, and dimming the lights at dusk. Since I had long eliminated caffeine (including one of my favorite foods, chocolate ice cream) and was avoiding stimulating activities, it was a matter of getting off screens after dinner and imposing more structure. If I could get myself out of bed in the morning, the rest wouldn't be too difficult.

I wasn't living alone, though. When David came home one evening with a stack of Reese Witherspoon DVDs, which meant he was desperate to watch *anything* with me, I said Reese would have to wait. "No screens at night, remember?" When I turned off all the lights at dusk and lit some candles, Rosa protested, "Too spooky, mama!" and switched them back on. To get around this, I ordered a pair of orange goggles to filter out the blue light, thereby tricking the brain into thinking it was actually dark. With them on, I looked like a fruit fly. (To this day, I turn into a fruit fly at dusk.) When I removed the digital clock from our bedroom so it wouldn't broadcast how many minutes I lay awake—which might prompt obsessive calculations of baseball games—David insisted on keeping the clock, to get him to work on time.

It would have been easier to move to the wilderness alone and let them live their lives. But since I couldn't do that, I moved to the living room couch. We only had the one bedroom, and Rosa was crammed in the fainting room.

"I thought you were trying to get *off* the couch," David said, unconvinced by this setup.

"Funny," I said. "At night I get to be on it."

I threw a sheet over the cushions, then tossed my comforter and pillow on top. The makeshift bed didn't look half bad. But as twilight came, the living room turned into an urban jungle. With my senses being hyper-efficient transducers of the energies around me, every noise and light felt like it was hooked up to amplifiers. The glow of the city through the skylights, the streetcar squealing as it climbed the hill behind our house, the pigeons cooing, the cars puttering around Dolores Park. I armored myself with an eye mask and a pair of earplugs.

A few weeks into my experiment, I moved back to sleeping in the bedroom and tried medication. I chose gentle drugs with fewer potential side effects, like Benadryl and Unisom. When those didn't work, I tried Ambien and Lunesta. Nothing touched my insomnia. My circadian clock, it seemed, was resistant to a reset.

My irritable mood broke through the cool politeness I had been maintaining, and small things started to trigger me.

"Have you tried melatonin?" David asked one day, hoping his suggestion might mitigate the situation.

"It's a supplement," I growled, "not a drug."

"What's the difference? Lots of people take it for jet lag."

"Drugs are drugs, and supplements are supplements. Supplements are 'alternative.'" I added some air quotes for emphasis. "They're not regulated like drugs are, so I'm leery of them—how can I know what I'm getting?"

It hadn't even dawned on me that I might be deficient in melatonin, and if so, I might be able to treat a *cause* of my sleep troubles—the very hypothesis of my named experiment. I was thinking of melatonin the way I thought of drugs—as something to manage my symptoms. I didn't know then that melatonin could impact the signaling to other hormones like stress hormones, as well as thyroid hormones. Or that melatonin could reduce inflammation and also affect the power generators of the cells, potentially improving fatigue.

One night, as the urban jungle started playing with my senses and I thought I was hearing howler monkeys in the distance, I went to the bathroom and opened the medicine cabinet for another eenie-meenie-miney-mo of which medicine to try. Next to the Benadryl was a small bottle I hadn't seen before. Made of blue glass, it looked like it came from a medieval apothecary. I picked it up and examined the label. MELATONIN ELIXIR. It had the whiff of Juan Carlos. He had been learning about Western supplements along with traditional Chinese herbs, and David must have asked him for recommendations. At almost two a.m., ready to pull my hair out, I couldn't have cared less if this was a tonic of bird saliva. I took two squirts.

When sleep didn't take me, I donned my goggles and opened *The Catcher in the Rye*. It was my third time reading this book, but my first time in orange. The narrator's rant of the world being ruled by phonies made me see a certain phoniness in my orange filters and synthetic elixirs correcting the effects of an artificial world. So I closed my eyes, yearning again for the naturalness of the African savanna. I don't know how much time passed, because I fell asleep! I got about five hours of continuous sleep that night. And while it wouldn't be a magic cure-all—nothing on this journey would be—the melatonin cracked the door open, little by little, to the new world of supplements.

For quality assurance, I learned that some companies test their products through independent third parties. There were *Consumer Reports*–type groups that screen products for safety and quality. And there were websites on the science of vitamins and supplements, including my go-to site for all things scientific, PubMed, a comprehensive database for the National Institutes of Health. The research had long been there, I just hadn't known about it.

Soon, I added magnesium to my nighttime regimen. An "essential" mineral—meaning the body can't produce it, so it has to be acquired through food, water, or supplements—magnesium is involved in hundreds of key chemical reactions in the body. Magnesium promotes relaxation and facilitates energy metabolism. It reduces inflammation and regulates sleep, too. Half of all Americans don't get enough magnesium through their diets. So repleting my magnesium levels was another example of treating the root cause instead of masking the symptoms.

In the coming weeks, I added chamomile tea, Epsom salt baths, and lavender essential oils. These homey remedies were also backed by science as having anti-inflammatory and anti-anxiety properties, along with low-risk profiles and long traditions of use. The combination of melatonin, magnesium, and the day-night hygiene measures was the start of regulating my body's rhythms and easing inflammation. Beyond the physical, I felt a hint of mental renewal: empowerment.

As I took my cocktail one night, David caught me in the bathroom. "What's that?"

"My sleep regimen—magnesium and melatonin."

He raised his eyebrows.

I raised mine back. "You look surprised."

"Well, you can be very...."

"Stubborn? I know."

I had long thought of my skepticism as my shield against untruth. But I realized now that it had been shielding me from undiscovered truths, too. Truths I might not readily embrace. Watching Rosa and Sonia navigate the world, I saw that their minds were open to all possibilities. They used their analytical minds to ask questions and gather answers systematically in their toddler ways, often coming up with "no, that's hot," or "no, that's scary," even when there wasn't physical proof. In their experiments were abundant yeses. This was the opposite of my "no way" attitude, which started out with "prove it to me," and ended with "prove it to me some more." To move the zipper *here*-ward, I had to learn to trust experience as enough. And to be open to being open itself.

In the meantime, I took more immediate gratification in noting the next step in my How to Get off the Couch assignment:

2. Reset your inner clock.

THIRTEEN

2009

The gains in sleep were up and down, but overall, up. My moods seemed more stable. But it was hard to tell where my overall energy was. If my thyroiditis days put me at 8–9 on the functionality scale and the time since the sudden disturbance in Beijing was 1–2, the attempt at circadian reset might have moved my zipper half a point, to 1.5–2.5. This meant I could leave the house a few times a week for an hour or two, and my symptoms remained moderate to severe.

The health and illness zipper continuum, I was learning, wasn't a straight line, but a corkscrew with *here* (health) at the summit, reached only after a painfully slow climb, and *there,* a swift slide to the bottom. As hard as I tried, I couldn't identify inciting triggers. And I worried constantly about setbacks. They happened a lot, and even when they didn't, the threat was always there, hovering.

I did my best to keep a daily routine. Having understood the science on the circadian clock, I believed it was in my best interest. If Rosa and Sonia did better on a schedule, why not do the same for myself? The payoff might come later, I reasoned, even if it was months away. There were times when I would break the rules, though—to sleep in whenever I could (with young children, this was rare), and to eat outside of structured meals. Because to keep my energy from falling and my nerves from triggering, I had to eat around the clock.

With things moving so slowly, the cool politeness in our marriage grew tedious. We were still tiptoeing around our issues instead of confronting them. Rosa would soon be starting preschool and we had a hard time collaborating on the application process, which in San Francisco was intensive. Placement included lengthy forms, mandatory interviews, and discussions of Rosa's goals and our goals for her. She was three and a half! When all was said and done, we received a formal acceptance letter in the mail, feeling like she had gotten into Harvard. The tuition felt that way, too.

"Are you okay with Rosa going to this school?" I asked David. "I mean, since you're paying for it and all."

"It's *our* money, Cynthia. Not *mine*."

"Really, it's not," I said under my breath.

I knew this passive aggression was maddening, but in the protracted coolness, I was tired of not speaking my truth. If a part of me was trying to provoke him, I got it right back.

"Do you have any idea..." he said, his words trailing off.

"Any idea of what?"

"Of when you might go back to work?"

So there it was. I had gotten him to say what I sensed he had been feeling all along: that he was tired of being the sole earner. It was the only logical conclusion I could draw, because he knew I was lucky to get out of the house at all, for an hour or two a day at best; and I knew we still had plenty in savings. I had felt like dead weight all along, too.

"I'll go back as soon as I can."

The next week, the cool politeness turned icy. When David asked me to pass the salt and pepper, I replied, "Don't worry, I'll go back as soon as I can." When he installed the new shower heads and asked how I liked them—months had passed since he had ordered them, but that's how hard it was to get non-essential tasks done—I replied, "Don't worry, I'll go back as soon as I can." There were no fights. Not even the hint of a fight. There were no emotions whatsoever.

Finally, David lifted the body pillow divider on our bed one night, as if giving me some air in my shoebox. "Just a couple."

"A couple what?"

"A couple sessions with a counselor."

A few weeks later, we met at a counselor's office in a historic mansion in the Pacific Heights district. It felt good to be out in the big world. Her office was airy, the ceilings vaulted and decorated with plaster ornaments. She sat down in a leather armchair facing a long window, her legs crossed, posture erect. Her speech was formal, but there was a warmth in her manner. Opposite her were two other armchairs, a few feet apart, where David and I sat. Close, but not touching.

"Can you tell me a bit about why you're here," she began, "and what you're hoping to get out of these sessions?"

David and I looked at each other, neither of us sure how to be open and direct with a total stranger. Given his strong dislike of therapy, I assumed I would be the first to talk. So while I was thinking how to best frame the situation, how to be direct but not too direct, concise but not too concise, David spoke up.

"We're here because most of our weeks are hard. Last week was no exception." He explained my health problems.

"Please don't blame it all on me." I rolled my eyes, not liking how he had opened things up. I would have preferred to start off with our backgrounds. "The issues we have are issues *any* couple has. Yes, my health issues make things worse. I can't work, I can't earn money, but we mostly fight about sex and social energy. Like if he goes out less often with his friends, or if we have less sex, it feels like it's all my fault. But a lot of this is simply the life stage we're in, isn't it?"

She acknowledged me, but said, "Please let David continue."

Taken aback, I fidgeted in my chair and tried to listen quietly.

She gets upset at me for the smallest things, I heard.

She wants things perfect around the house.

She gets mad at me for not helping out.

She doesn't see how much I have to deal with.

She seems to want to make me suffer because she's suffering. The whole thing with her health is so unpredictable—her moods, her symptoms, her energy.

My stomach was knotting up. Now it was my turn.

He doesn't hear me until *after* I get upset and by then I've already tried dozens of times to communicate calmly.

He only sees the anger itself and not the reason for the anger.

He always sees what I *don't* do, not all that I *do* do, and of course it's much less than if I felt a hundred percent.

He pretends like life is normal, and maybe his is, but mine isn't.

She took a moment to gather her thoughts. "What I hear are two main areas of stress. David has a hard time confronting anger. And Cynthia feels dismissed."

We nodded simultaneously.

She asked us to dig into our childhoods for the earliest memories of our respective challenges—his confronting anger, mine with dismissal.

"I was such a sensitive child, so I felt dismissed a lot," I said. "Probably even when people didn't mean to dismiss me." I recounted the episode of the roly-poly sanctuary in which the very bugs I was trying to save had died, how guilty I felt, how stupid I felt, and how my family laughed.

The counselor simply listened, as did David. I felt unexpectedly moved, as if having a witness for the parts of myself I had long been ashamed of was healing in and of itself. After this moment of silent recognition, she looked to David.

"There was a time in middle school when I got a bad report card," he said. He started cracking his knuckles, one after the other, and I knew that this process was excruciating for him. "My mother got really angry. It was more her facial expression than her words...and maybe it was just *her* more than her facial expression. My mother and father—they're each so accomplished in their fields. They've always been so work-focused and focused on making a contribution to the world. I guess I was afraid. Afraid I had let her down."

I could see David not as Superman, but as a mere mortal. I wondered if he had felt Number Two to his mother and father, and to the implicit expectation that he would make a significant contribution to the world, beyond being a good person—the expectation of being a good person who did great things. I felt a tenderness toward him. Suddenly it felt strange to be sitting close to him and not touching.

"Each time you argue," the counselor said, "these formative experiences and the emotions they arouse are the real issues. The root issues. Disagreements happen between all couples. But the heat is often only a symptom of unresolved stresses, many seeded in childhood, more than the issues on the surface. So if you can identify and address the roots, the heat in your fights—the symptoms—will likely lessen, or better yet, vanish all together."

The root issues, I noted in my pocket journal. *The heat is often only a symptom.*

On the ride back, we drove with the windows down, fresh air against my face.

Back in my small world, Sonia leapt into my arms as Ayi said goodbye. Having used up my energy with the counseling session, I put Sonia down and wondered how I would make dinner or give the girls a bath. I decided instead to head straight for the couch. But I was too late. David had already assumed the role of a lava monster and the girls were squealing to and fro, leaping from couch cushion to couch cushion, my beloved refuge now engulfed by a sea of lava. I went to the fainting room to find it a cluttered mess. I retreated to the bedroom, only to hear the neighbor to our left, whose living room walls abutted our bedroom, blaring what sounded like Miley Cyrus on steroids. Then Sonia began to cry. The walls of our crowded flat seemed to be closing in. There was nowhere to go!

I longed for David to stop playing for one second, to either offer Sonia some milk without my having to ask, or to pause his roughhousing. The tenderness I felt in the counseling session was giving way to a long-seeded resentment. Okay, I huffed, trying to convince myself that these weren't the *real* issues. How was this related to the roly-polies again? In the moment, I couldn't see the connection. These tensions felt real and ever-present.

It was fatigue rather than insight that kept me from intervening in the living room. The fatigue forced me to do nothing and wait it out. To my relief, after ten minutes or so, the living room became peaceful. And to my surprise, the music next door finished its run, too. In the quietude, I closed my eyes and tried to recall the counseling session as it happened. How I had seen a vulnerable side of David. How we had gone into some darker experiences together. How I had finally felt seen around the roly-poly incident, and how the early imprints of feeling invisible might be fueling the intensity of feeling unseen by David now. I replayed the counselor's departing words: Identify the root issues. The heat is often only a symptom.

Trying to extrapolate this idea into a larger concept of health, I returned to my *Pathologic Basis of Disease* textbook and reviewed the mechanisms of disease. If heat was only a symptom and heat was inflammation, and if, as I had recently learned, the body didn't discriminate between physical and emotional stresses, could it be that the inflammation in my body wasn't the primary culprit per se, and there were deeper root causes or experiences fueling it? It made sense as I pondered it now. This was a sophisticated way to restate and approach my original hypothesis.

Clearer, I left the bedroom and checked out the scene in the kitchen. During my brief intermission, Juan Carlos had popped upstairs to help David, and together they were making a late dinner. The girls were unbathed but happily engrossed in a *Dora the Explorer* video. The fatigue that had forced me to do nothing and relinquish control was allowing others to step up. It was forcing me to say *Yes, I can be tended to without guilt* and *Yes, I can do nothing even if others are doing, doing, doing.*

As the streetcar screeched along the tracks behind our house, I glanced at the clock. The train was a few minutes behind schedule, but showing up nonetheless. "Frittata's in the oven," David said. Before I could say a word of thanks, he added, "And I'll run a bath for the girls."

3. Give yourself permission to receive.

FOURTEEN

The next week, I was laid out on the couch for five days. Why, I couldn't pinpoint. Autoimmunity was just this way. We had to postpone our second counseling session, and I had to miss Rosa's first day at preschool. David dropped her off with a backpack and an extra change of clothes, in case of accidents. He assured me it wasn't a big deal that I missed it; the teachers only allowed curbside drop-offs anyhow, to ease separation anxiety. Okay, I said, reminding myself of 3: *Give yourself permission to receive.* I was trying to receive David's gesture of taking our daughter to school, but I couldn't figure out what else I was supposed to gain. Letting go felt like I was ceding what little possession I had of my life.

To repossess my life, I knew I had to deal with the day-to-day noise and claustrophobia of our urban flat. Constant noise was a problem for my hypersensitive ears. But it wasn't until I researched the basics that I learned the term *noise pollution.* It was a major public health issue, one the World Health Organization ranked as second to air pollution in terms of health risks. Noise pollution activates the fight-or-flight nervous system. Since healing requires people to be in the rest-and-digest state, noise pollution can impede healing. And being stuck in fight-or-flight is, in fact, a cause of immune dysfunction and inflammation. Even noise that isn't consciously registered, like traffic sounds in the background or dogs barking while people slept, can cause stress responses to rise, and hence, inflammation to rise.

I decided to make quietness a priority, not just a preference. There weren't many green or natural spaces near our house that could be characterized as serene, so I sought out a church. St. Anne's, the pink church from my old hood, was too far away now. But the Mission Dolores church was two city blocks away. Between Mass and confessional hours, it was perfectly empty. I would sit in the back pew and gaze upon the vaulted ceiling, stealing glances at the crucifix. I couldn't look at the suffering Christ for long, because my brokenness would feel all the more apparent, which would defeat the purpose of a sanctuary. Instead, I focused on the in-between spaces—the shadows of the pews, the hollows of the arches—and found peace there. On occasion, a middle-aged man would come in and sit toward the front, recite a few prayers in Spanish, then leave. Kurt's energy wasn't there, as it used to be in empty churches. If I pictured anyone sitting next to me, it was David. I wished he would sometimes leave his doing-ness behind and just *be* with me.

Over a few visits to Mission Dolores, I began to notice how my shoulders would relax and my heart would slow down. One day, I brought along my Timex wristwatch and blood pressure cuff and measured the time it took my body to reach the rest-and-digest state— roughly forty-five minutes. Three quarters of an hour of doing nothing in a sanctuary to get my nervous system calmed down! This kind of impaired capacity of the nervous system to shut down the stress response was common in patients with chronic fatigue. Over time, I would compare my vital sign measurements, finding that my nervous system was trainable. The more often I sat in the sanctuary, the quicker I could reach rest-and-digest. Three months later, it would only take twenty-two minutes.

Seeking rest-and-digest in our marriage, too, David and I attended a second counseling session. This time, we kept things more practical, hoping to figure out, with the counselor's guidance, how to fight better. She gave us useful tips, like listening before talking, using *I* statements over *you* statements, and avoiding words like *always* and *never*. It wasn't anything revolutionary, but getting a refresher course was helpful. One new suggestion we especially appreciated was to find neutral ground— to explore places that were new to us as a couple. A change of scenery could bring us to a different mindset, which might help break unhealthy patterns.

After the session ended, David committed to putting these techniques into practice. But he also reminded me that he had fulfilled the "couple of sessions" he had offered, and that he was done. Though I would have preferred to continue, his decision was fine by me. Applying these practical strategies and delving into my past gave me a lifetime's worth of assignments.

A few weeks later, on a Saturday, David proposed a fresh outing. His cousin John was starring in a play in Emeryville, across the bay, and was holding tickets for us at will call. David had arranged for his parents to babysit Rosa and Sonia. *A date?* My malaise and dizziness were as tame as they could be in those days, and I couldn't remember when I had last dared to consider a real outing for us.

David started packing Sonia's diaper bag. "All you have to do is sit there, both in the car and at the play."

My mental bookkeeper went through her usual calculations on energy saved and energy spent, how I would fare, and whether I would pay for it tomorrow. I wanted to go, I didn't want to go.

David grew restless. "If we're gonna go, we need to leave now, in case there's traffic. Look, I'll drive, and I'll drop you off at the door."

Before the reflexive "no" could slip out of my mouth, an inner voice reminded me of 3: *Give yourself permission to receive.* So, bypassing my mental bookkeeper, who always played it safe, I blurted, "Okay."

He paused, looking stunned at the relatively minimal amount of resistance I gave him, then finished packing the diaper bag. I asked him to get the girls ready, as I went to the bedroom. I needed ten or fifteen minutes.

"You don't need to make yourself up," he said. "You look great."

I wasn't worried in the least about my hair or makeup. I simply needed to get out of my sweats. Despite his living with me and seeing my health challenges up close, David still had no idea how far I was from doing things spontaneously like I used to. Just pick up and go was no longer something I could do. To undress, I still had to break down the motions like a puppeteer, *Left foot first, steady, pull pant leg off. Okay, now right foot.* I thought I was moving quickly until David began to tap the car horn, and I was still standing in my underwear. After getting dressed, I drank a glass of salty water to prevent worsening dizziness. In sloth time, I made it to the car.

On the Bay Bridge, the big world looked surreal, like I was revisiting the past. The fast cars ahead. The cargo ships below. I rolled the window down and closed my eyes to really feel the ocean breeze on my cheeks, a slight residue of salt in my hair. *This isn't the past,* I had to remind myself. *This is me, now.*

Traffic turned out to be light. With an extra hour to kill, David suggested we explore a place that was new to me—his childhood neighborhood in Berkeley, the next town over from Emeryville. At a dead end on the north side of Virginia Street stood a tall, brown-shingled apartment house. David pulled over and pointed out the corner unit. That was where his mother had worked on her dissertation, he said, and where he kept her company as a baby. We stepped out, picked a few loquats from an old tree, and then David suggested we drive deeper into the neighborhood. We meandered through narrow, quirky streets, past a rambling creek, a pocket park, and the city rose garden. On a quiet street with a peek-a-boo view, we parked and watched the sun set over the Golden Gate Bridge. It was reminiscent of the days when we had traveled without any agenda.

Fifteen minutes passed. A man walked out from the adjacent house. He was middle-age, tall and slender, and dressed in plaid flannel. His hair was reddish-brown, thinning on top.

"Gorgeous view," David said.

Saying nothing, the man went about his business shoveling wood chips and digging a hole in the front yard. He rested his shovel and lifted his eyes, which were somber. "I've lived here for more than fifty years," he said. "I grew up in this house, and every single sunset has been different." He seemed to be talking more to himself than to us. Then he went to the garage, took out a For Sale sign, and pounded it into the hole.

"It must be amazing to watch the sun set every day," I said.

He didn't say anything in response. Instead, seemingly out of nowhere, he invited us to see his house. The economy had recently fallen into a recession, and we later learned that the house had sat on the market for four months with no offers, which was unheard of in the Bay Area. He was desperate to show the house to anyone, even random passersby like us. And out of curiosity, we said "Sure."

The house was a hundred-year-old, brown-shingled lodge. Paneled in wood, the living areas smelled like an old forest. The floors were warped, causing a downward slope to the entire lower level. There were also old-timey accents like clinker brick hearths, a hand-crank fire alarm, a latched window screen for milk deliveries, and a pre-digital "intercom"—a plastic tube in the wall that connected the first and second floors.

As we walked around, I could tell by David's face and posture that he was taken by the house. We had outgrown our flat, but we had never talked about moving, and certainly not out of the city, away from his parents, Juan Carlos, and Ayi. And with David's recent question about when I might return to work, I was surprised at his interest. Besides, something about the house was off. There was a staleness, not in the air but in the house itself. Like the gravity of life was too much for it to hold up. It felt depressed.

My reservations started to fade when I stepped into the backyard. It was a slice of Eden. Not in the way of perfection, but of wildness. The lot was long. Old garden beds lined the gravel paths, which were over-grown with sour grass, miner's lettuce, and wild onions. I ambled into the weeds and came to a weeping cypress. Its crown had been lopped off to open the view for an uphill neighbor. Hanging on its trunk was a tattered hammock. I lay on it, sinking the weight of my body into its hold, staring up at the cypress from its underside. In a much shorter time than forty-five minutes—it had to be less than fifteen, since we had to get on our way to the play—I felt my breath relax and my heart rate slow down. Rest-and-digest came much faster in this sanctuary of wood and leaves. I found myself thinking, *I can live in the backyard.*

At intermission during the play, David said, "What do you think?"

I sipped some bubbly water. "Your cousin's great in this role."

"I mean about the house."

"The yard is magical. But I thought you were worried about living within our means."

He took out his phone and started surfing the Internet. It turned out that it was 10 percent cheaper to live in Berkeley than in San Francisco, and the preschools were considerably more affordable. After some mental calculations, before I could even finish my bubbly water and pretzels, we had agreed to submit an offer. It was crazy, but it took us back to a time when life was novel, and reclaimed for us a sense of agency over our lives. Grateful, I squeezed David's hand. We could raise the girls with more space, closer to nature, in a pace slower than San Francisco's, where I might have a better chance to heal, and return to work sooner.

Three days later, our offer was accepted.

The house needed a facelift and some leveling. To assess the problem of the floors, David hired a skilled young contractor named Zac Bischoff. Zac had studied architecture and engineering, weaving together art and science in his work. It was apparent in the way he surveyed the house with David and me, measuring problem areas with lasers and marking them with blue tape to indicate which parts needed lifting and by how much—but careful not to be hasty. The process of lifting the house would take about a week, he explained. One day, I watched him in the basement, jacking up the foundation by a couple of millimeters, like he was jacking up a car.

"How do you know when to stop?" I asked.

"You're a doctor, so you know bones," he said, with a slight drawl. "The bones of this old house are like the bones of an old woman." He stroked his palm along a timber beam. "If you raise her too quickly or make her too straight, she's prone to break. So the key is to listen and feel for creaks. Then, just before she cracks, you stop. Even if the measurements aren't perfect."

Zac approached this house as an n of 1, evaluating it as an individual case. Over the coming months, whenever I could make a trip to the house with David, I would pay close attention to Zac's methodology. Our century-old house had irregular floorboards and wood panels that weren't standardized; Zac would find or invent ways to accommodate them. If he opened up a wall and found unexpected pipes connected to nothing, or old-fashioned features whose purposes weren't clear, he would always say, "Not a problem, we'll work around them." His end-goal was rarely a precise measurement. Function mattered more than numbers.

Before I left the house, I would take time to sit under the weeping cypress, or stroll around the backyard, wondering how the beehives would do here, wondering where I might sleep, perhaps under the stars. After several visits, I was clear on one thing, that my body consistently felt less inflamed and less revved up here.

One evening, I looked up the science, to understand why I felt better in nature. Study after study showed that green spaces shifted the autonomic nervous system from fight-or-flight to rest-and-digest. Consequently, moods, blood pressure, heart rate, and breathing patterns improved, and stress hormone levels decreased. Short doses of nature, including mere photographs of nature, sharpened performance. Other studies showed they increased feelings of generosity and social connectedness. The presence of houseplants in hospital rooms lessened pain and hastened recovery from surgery. Studies of functional brain scans showed regions associated with empathy and love lighting up when exposed to nature scenes, while urban scenes and sounds lit up regions associated with fear and anxiety.

I added my next entry to the How to Get Off the Couch list:

4. Get a daily dose of nature.

Not wanting to delay this until our move, I asked David to pick up some new houseplants, two at a time, until each room had a couple. I sat under the plum tree on the back deck for increasingly longer periods of time, and on sunnier days, ate breakfast and lunch there with the girls. Once, as I was taking my daily dose of nature, a shadow flew into my line of sight. A green hummingbird. Sapphire head, green bodice, a blotch of red on the chest.

"Look, girls!" I whispered. Their eyes widened. We watched the bird flit about, darting between us and the plum tree, back and forth, back and forth, within an arm's reach, his coal eyes fixed on us.

"He's saying, 'Lightly, lightly,'" Rosa whispered.

"Yes, that's what it seems like his wings are saying."

"No, Mama, he's talking. Can't you hear him?"

I could feel the breeze from his wings, and felt like I could practically pluck a feather from his tail—but no, I couldn't hear him, and I wouldn't ever hear him, because the voice was a figment of Rosa's wild imagination. That's what I believed then. In hindsight, however, I'm not sure what I believe about that episode. Because my corkscrew journey would soon take a sudden and unexpected turn, and life as I knew it would become strange, and stranger yet, until my whole worldview of what was possible would change forever.

FIFTEEN

The house renovations continued. David took Rosa to England for a friend's wedding, and I had some time alone with Sonia. I was getting my daily doses of nature, taking my Epsom salts baths, wearing my orange goggles, taking my thyroid medication and melatonin and magnesium, continuing my training of the circadian clock, practicing letting go and receiving, and drinking my salty water. As I think about them now, these tasks weren't a big deal. But for someone who wasn't used to taking care of herself or putting herself at Number One, they felt like a full-time job.

Though my energy was still slow to increase, other symptoms began to vanish, subtly, and largely realized in hindsight. Like the need to eat around the clock—now, after dinner, a small snack could tide me over until morning. And the need to urinate—it was now every two or three hours instead of every hour, which helped me sleep longer, too.

With David and Rosa gone, I tried to figure out how to entertain Sonia. She was almost two, and seemed to have the vigor of three toddlers. We would watch the dogs run on the hill, and Sonia would jump off my lap and chase them around, thankfully burning a lot of her energy. When I couldn't get off the couch, she would jump on our bed like a trampoline, and tumble on the mat in our living room. With her toddlerhood in full bloom, her golden joy could explode into a crimson rage in a matter of seconds. Besides the dogs, there were only two things known to soothe her: *The Backyardigans* cartoons and baking. I used both activities, often.

The day of our banana nut loaf experiment was when things started getting weird. The phone rang, I didn't feel like taking any calls, and no message was left on the answering machine. It rang a second time, then a third. What-ifs stirred in my mind, various scenarios of family emergencies, so I finally decided to pick up.

"Cynthia?" asked a cheerful voice.

"Yes," I said, unable to place it.

"It's Pia. It's been too long. I just wanted to see how everything's going. Are you all right?" Pia was the clairvoyant friend I had met through David, the one he had suggested I call during my difficult pregnancy (which I had not done).

"I suppose things are okay." My mind was on Sonia, whose hands were in the clumpy batter. "Um," I said, redirecting my focus to Pia, "there's been a lot going on. We bought a house in Berkeley, and we're doing renovations on it, and trying to get Rosa into a new preschool after all the trouble of getting her into one here in the city… Let's see, what else can I tell you?"

As I was thinking, there was a long silence on the other end. An eerie feeling came over me, as I realized Pia might be reading me like a crystal ball. Having only ever heard stories about her gifts, I had never directly experienced them. I liked Pia, and found her a compassionate, if not a very reasonable, person. But in church as a young girl, I had heard the pastor and Sunday-school teachers warn against such people, that they were witches, and their deeds were evil. This left me spooked. Why was she calling now?

"You've been putting out some distress signals," she said, still cheerful.

I looked at my hands, covered in flour, and wondered what she was picking up. I had no idea how to answer such a statement.

"You still there?" Pia said.

"Yeah, still here." I washed our hands and put the banana nut loaf in the oven.

Pia continued, saying I had been "reaching out" energetically for days, so she had sat with my image in meditation, to see what came up. "Oranges," she said. "Tons of oranges flying around!"

"Oranges?" I said.

"Does that mean anything to you?"

"Vitamin C, maybe? You know, I've been having a lot of health challenges."

"Ah," she said, "that's what the distress signals were about."

She said she had also seen carpets.

Carpets? I had just relocated from the kitchen to the bedroom, where I was now glancing at the beige carpet below my feet. I began to scan the windows, the ceiling, the closet, the whole room, wondering what she saw.

She mumble-whispered, as though talking to herself. "Maybe something in the carpet…it's nothing to get worried about. Just some chemicals to remove."

Before I dared to ask any questions—I was more preoccupied about the source of her information than the content of it—she had switched to mundane matters: how she and her husband, Don, were doing; how their grandchildren were growing up; how Don's daughter lived in the Bay Area; and how they would love to see us the next time they visited.

The restraint in my voice (or perhaps it was the energy I was emitting?) might have told her I was uncomfortable, because before we said good-bye, she said, "This energy stuff can be unsettling at first, but I'm just tuning into what already *is*."

I wondered if she was hallucinating, or if she had any history of mental illness. It would have been more reassuring to me than the possibility that she was tapping into an alternate reality.

I said thanks, and that we would love to see them, then hung up the phone. The call left me unsettled, and before it got too late in England, I called David.

He found my story fascinating.

"You don't think it's freaky?" I asked.

"Freaky is fascinating. Besides, I want you to feel better. If Pia saw an infection in someone else's hip, maybe she can see something that would help with your health, too."

I held the receiver back and glared at it with astonishment. Perhaps he didn't care where his information came from. But the Truth with a capital "T" mattered to me. And what Pia did just didn't fit into that.

The next week, David and Rosa returned with stories of the English wedding, a visit to Buckingham Palace, and Madame Tussauds Wax Museum. As the jet-lagged two slept in late, I was preparing breakfast for Sonia and myself when, suddenly, Pia's voice echoed in my mind as if I was talking to her. *Oranges.* I caught my hands mid-action: I was peeling an orange! I shook my head a few times, trying to quiet the voice. I wanted to think I was too rational to be influenced by her visions, but they had a power over me. I ate a slice, then two. I also took a hefty dose of vitamin C, in case that was what the oranges symbolized. Later that day, Pia's voice echoed again as I walked from room to room, keenly aware of the carpet. I tramped over that carpet, straight to my laptop.

I searched online for "chemicals in carpets." Blogs and news headlines with the word *toxic* filled the page. I was blown away. *This benign, inert-appearing carpet?* I clicked on an article from *The New York Times Magazine*—a balanced, well-researched voice of reason. The journalist wrote of everyday chemicals lurking in our homes. But two words in particular caught my eye: *breast milk.* According to the article, harmful indoor chemicals had been measured in the urine, fat, blood, and breast milk of the majority of Americans tested. In *my* breast milk? I wondered.

I kept reading. Flame retardants on couches. Additives in skin lotions. Nonstick coating on pans. Plastics in baby bottles. Much of it associated with infertility, diabetes, obesity, cancer…*and thyroid disorders.* These chemicals were called "endocrine disruptors," meaning they interfere with the intricate web of hormones and their functioning.

Unsure what to make of this, I went to my go-to science database, PubMed, and searched for "endocrine disruptors." More than a thousand articles came up. Sifting through the abstracts, I learned just how many everyday, legal chemicals made people sick, often by disrupting their hormones. Had these chemicals caused some of my health problems? Was Pia right about the very carpet under my toes?

I thought about the perfumes I wore in high school, seeping into my skin.

All the lotions, shampoos, deodorants, and makeup.

The plastics I microwaved food in.

The herbicides and pesticides on my foods—literally, having chemicals for breakfast, lunch, and dinner.

The paints and nail polish and other solvents I inhaled.

The aerosolized chemicals from all the couches I ever sat on.

The formaldehyde vapors from my cadaver in medical school.

The industrial bleaches in the hospitals.

The air pollution in Beijing.

The thyroid gland was one of the most sensitive tissues with regard to pollutants. Pesticides, herbicides, nonstick cookware, and plastics in canned foods and water bottles could disrupt the signaling of and to the thyroid gland. Other pollutants, like a contaminant from rocket fuel that leaches into the water supply and gets absorbed by leafy vegetables, could inhibit the thyroid's production of hormones. Flame retardants, certain byproducts of coal, and additives in lubricants could trigger autoimmune reactions against the thyroid (Hashimoto's). It dawned on me that thyroid medications had been among the most commonly prescribed drugs in America for years. Could this be explained, in part, by the explosion of these chemicals?

My poor thyroid, I thought. By limiting exposures to such chemicals, I wasn't expecting to see health improvements right away, but it might prevent my health from worsening. In theory, it would also protect David's health and the girls'. The girls! When I thought of exposing them to invisible chemicals, a fierceness welled up in me, a mama bear intent on protecting her cubs. I went straight to the kitchen, where a nonstick pan was on the stove. It was time to clean house.

I tossed out the nonstick pan. Garbage.

Then a worn plastic ladle.

Two plastic water bottles. Into the recycling bin.

David entered. "Whoa, why are you throwing out perfectly good things?"

"I'm protecting our family."

"From what?"

"Poisons lurking in our stuff."

He might have judged me as paranoid, but my actions were based in hard science. Rational thought mattered more than ever, as I was keenly aware of having arrived at this information by way of Pia's visions. While reducing harmful chemicals could detoxify the house, there was also the matter of detoxifying the body. I wouldn't know this until years later, but detoxification—the body's innate capacity to remove toxic substances that build up, generate inflammation, and contribute to disease—can be optimized and personalized. For now, detoxifying the house was a big enough undertaking, and it took a good part of the afternoon to rummage through the rest of the cabinets. By the end, the recycling bin was full and I was back on the couch.

I wondered how I hadn't known this before. When I had graduated from medical school, I had the impression that our primary defenses— the skin, respiratory tracts, and digestive tract—were complete barriers, only letting molecules pass selectively and intentionally. Now I wasn't so sure. Endocrine disruptors clearly entered our bodies without our permission or knowledge. Really, anything we put into the air, water, and earth ended up in us, and vice versa. It was also clear that, while cleaning house might reduce the amount of toxins my family was exposed to, this was only a stopgap solution. The items I threw out or recycled would end up somewhere else, and in someone else. As it was with health and illness, there was no *here/there* line between humans and the environment.

Healthy planet, healthy people.

Sick planet, sick people.

The information on harmful chemicals was new to me, but it wasn't new. There was a whole field supporting research and policies on healthier alternatives for everyday chemicals. Environmental health advocates honored the Precautionary Principle, which urges precaution in introducing chemicals until the weight of the evidence demonstrates their safety. Most chemicals weren't adequately tested for, and environmental regulations were outdated. They were based on toxicology models relying on the theory that "the dose makes the poison," meaning the higher the dose of the poison, the worse the health effects. But the problem with the newer hormone-disrupting chemicals was that they exerted effects at high levels...*and low levels*. The effects at these disparate levels could also differ. To figure out what others were doing about this public health crisis, and to find out if I could do anything, too, even if just from my couch, I joined a grassroots group, the Collaborative on Health and the Environment. They hosted free podcasts I could tune into, no matter what my condition.

The first live presentation I dialed into was "The Ecological Paradigm of Health," led by Harvard-trained public health doctor Ted Schettler. He explained how an ecosystem becomes healthy or sick: individual factors usually make small impacts, but multiple, dynamic factors acting together can either build resilience or cause harm. For example, a grassland experiencing hotter than average temperatures might maintain its general landscape. But what if it experiences hotter than average temperatures, invasion by non-native plants, and a hefty application of herbicides? The presentation concluded with a brief Q&A, during which I dialed in with a question. "How do you know which factors are causing what," I asked Dr. Schettler, "and how do you know which interventions are working, if so many are happening at once?"

"You can't really decipher one cause, one effect," he said.

"But in medicine"—*and for myself*, I thought—"I want to measure specific causes with specific effects."

"In systems thinking, what matters are the *interactions* between different factors, and these interactions are more synergistic than additive. The other important factor is timing. In people and animals, early life influences play a very significant role, as if programming your genes for later times in life. So with all this, there will always be an element of uncertainty."

In medicine, we were always searching for certainty, which reassured doctors and patients alike. Perhaps the role of a doctor, though, wasn't to declare certainty, but to say what we knew and to acknowledge some honest don't-knows, can't-knows, and wish-we-could-knows.

The body, I realized, wasn't a three-dimensional puzzle to be solved. It was a living, dynamic ecosystem to be nurtured. That's what made the Ecological Paradigm of Health so pivotal. It was a framework—observable and measurable—that could be used for complex, living systems. Instead of asking whether x causes y, or one cause for one effect, its strength was in observing what happens when x and y and z—throw in q, too—interact within a particular system across a certain period of time. This was a concrete paradigm that accounted for life's messy variables, precisely because of the element of uncertainty, and this paradigm could be applied to a rain forest, a desert, or the terrain of the human body.

Tying this back to *Pathologic Basis of Disease* and my hypothesis, I had learned that chronic disease was due to imbalances starting years before symptoms started or a diagnosis could be made, and that these imbalances led to chronic inflammation, often widespread. Now, with the Ecological Paradigm of Health, I was learning that chronic inflammation was likely due to multiple stresses interacting with each other, and their effects could be synergistic. It was possible, then, that by removing multiple stresses, the healing process might be synergistic, too.

In the coming months, this newfound knowledge would seep into my consciousness the way pollutants seep into the soil—slowly, and taking up residence for the long-term.

5. Detoxify the house.

SIXTEEN

2010

The renovations complete, we moved to Berkeley on the scheduled day. Well, our stuff moved anyway. David, the girls, and I were delayed by a week because of something that wasn't scheduled—a setback that put me in the ER again. During the weeks prior to the move, I had been pacing myself on the packing and sorting. Apparently, it wasn't enough. On the night before the move, my muscles cramped up, then twitched, and my whole body felt beaten to a pulp. An hour later, the undertow sensation, which I hadn't experienced in two years, began to pull at me from within, and I felt like I was on the verge of drowning into myself.

David was on a flight back from Southern California when this happened. Home alone with the girls and panicked, I called Ayi to watch them, called David's mother to meet me at the ER, then called 911. After some valium, an IV bolus of three liters of saline, and a panel of standard emergency tests—which all came back normal—I was discharged. It was all par for the course for dysautonomia and chronic fatigue syndrome. My discharge diagnoses: dehydration and "abnormal involuntary movements." The ER doctors had to call it *something*.

The next morning, David met with our "movers," a motley crew of friends and family, while I settled into his parents' house. After the furniture and boxes were moved over, David treated the crew to Cheeseboard pizza and homemade honey lemonade. He recounted this story to me when he returned to his parents' house that night. I was lying in his childhood bed in his old room, wearing a pair of navy cotton pajamas that were hanging in his closet. The room was dark, and David appeared haloed against the backlit hallway. I saw, perhaps for the first time, his saintliness and all he had been carrying.

"Thank you for all you do, sweetheart," I whispered, not having the strength to talk. "I'm so sorry I couldn't help today."

David wept.

I convalesced in his childhood bed for a week, until I was strong enough to sit in a car. This ER visit, which would be my last, was another turning point for David and me. On our new foundation of counseling sessions, strengthened by the outing to the play and the joint decision to buy the house and create a new home together, we had been slowly reshaping our marriage. There was a sense of the future, something I had lost when Kurt had died.

The ER visit jolted me out of the languishing pattern of fatigue, into a clearer desire for life. More than an act of steel mental will, I uncovered a heart-based desire to live—not in the generic sense, but to live *my* life, the one in front of me, bruised muscles and confused inner workings and all. So when the four of us rode over to the new house a week later, even as the ocean breeze was too stimulating for me and I couldn't tolerate the traffic noise, I held David's hand and felt love, not fear, connecting us. Crossing the Bay Bridge, I found myself praying silently, *Thank you, Whoever Is There.*

The clarity of desire for my life spilled over to my life with David. An intact family wasn't just something I didn't want to lose, it was something I now wanted to nurture. No more passivity. No more crawling into existential shoeboxes for safety. Healing was a proactive mindset.

David arranged to work from home for a couple of weeks, until I got more stable. We talked about how to get the support we needed for the coming months. David's parents were now across the bay, as were our on-call friends, and Ayi couldn't do the long commute. The only other people I really considered were my parents. "But they're in Beijing," I said to David. "Besides, for the Chinese, the adult children take care of their parents, not the other way around, and they certainly don't burden their parents if they can help it."

"I'm finally learning that you have a hard time asking for you what you want," David said. "So, what do you *need*?"

"I need my mom and dad," I said without a moment's hesitation.

"Then let's call them."

Two weeks later, my parents arrived with four large suitcases and offered to stay for three generous months. My father had given up teaching a business ethics class at Beijing University, along with his work in the local church. My mother had left her Christian women's groups and church-sponsored service projects like orphanages for children with special needs.

I showed them the bedroom at the end of the hall, which was bare except for a bed and dresser. They dusted and vacuumed the room, unpacked their bags, rolled out an area rug, assembled two nightstands, and set up a vase with wildflowers my mother picked from the yard. Within a day, they had a pop-up guest room. They would soon turn to the rest of the house and do the same. David taught my father to use the electric drill, and my father went to task with blinds, curtains, bathroom accessories. My mother took up the frying pan and the grocery shopping, preparing two Chinese dishes every night, colorful and varied.

I pitched in whenever I could. If my parents were worried in any way about my condition, they didn't say. David was worried, though. Given my setback during the packing process, he urged me not to overdo it. He kept telling me Berkeley would be good for my health and he hoped I would be happier here. I think he was happier, too. He would kiss me good-bye and not ask any leading questions like, "What are you gonna do today?" I finally felt I had permission to relax. Soon, I found my favorite spot in the house, which I called "my perch"—and it wasn't the couch. It was a bay window seating area that looked onto the weeping cypress, a soft landing from which to watch the birds and the sunsets and the big world out yonder.

With this loving support and the space, the quiet, and the fifteen-degrees-warmer temperature than San Francisco, my nervous system seemed to be building some staying power in the rest-and-digest state, and showing a stronger capacity to bounce back. In a matter of weeks, not months, I would return to 2.0–2.5 on the functionality scale. Not captured on the scale was a notable increase in my trust in my healing experiment.

Sonia didn't seem happy with the relocation. During her afternoon naps, she would kick and scream and cling to me. Her solid little body was stronger than mine, and I was powerless to contain her. Photos of puppy dogs didn't work anymore; singing *The Backyardigans* theme song didn't either.

"This is our new home," I would say. "It's a nice place. You'll get used to it."

But she continued to refuse her afternoon naps. Worse, she would awaken around two or three a.m. with bloodcurdling cries. I had learned of night terrors during my pediatrics rotation. It was thought to be a passing phase, not usually a cause for concern. But Sonia's night terrors were a concern for me. My sleep was still tenuous at best and required strict hygiene measures.

Two weeks passed with her night terrors every night. Then she caught a bad cold from Rosa, who was bringing back a garden variety of germs from preschool, and in Sonia they triggered wheezing, and then she developed an angry rash around her lips that was resistant to salves or creams.

Why were all these things were happening at once?

"It's a phase lots of toddlers go through," the pediatrician said, when we brought Sonia in for an exam.

"I understand about night terrors," I said, "but is there anything we can do?"

"She just has to outgrow them."

"But what causes the terrors? And how long will they last?"

"They're like nightmares. The course varies from child to child."

"And what about her rash?" I said, hoping for a more tangible solution to a more tangible problem.

"Perioral dermatitis," she said. "It's a difficult rash to treat. You can try a topical steroid, but it doesn't seem to work as well as it does for other kinds of rashes."

"And the asthma?"

"I'm afraid we'll have to address that at another visit."

Steroids were the last thing I wanted on my daughter, and it would merely suppress her symptoms anyhow. I wanted to know *why*, and treat the causes. As the pediatrician typed in her electronic chart, I thought about the Ecological Paradigm of Health. If Sonia's body was an ecosystem, what cluster of disturbances might be causing the night terrors, the rash, and the asthma? Were they related in some way, since they occurred around the same time? I didn't understand how to put it all together.

We left the pediatrician's office with that familiar feeling of having run up against the limitations of medical care, and a doctor who didn't have the time to investigate beyond those limitations.

At night, I slept with Sonia to comfort her. I didn't get much sleep this way, and during my wakefulness, I noted something peculiar about Rosa, too: she would toss and turn and kick, sometimes violently, as though karate-chopping her mattress, and from time to time, she would awaken, complaining of pain along her shins. In the past, I might have written off these random symptoms as idiosyncratic or nothing serious. But knowing now that diseases start years or decades earlier as subtle imbalances, I decided to keep an eye on Rosa, too.

The following weekend, David and I hosted a potluck brunch to meet our neighbors. We wanted to know the folks who, without their knowing, were my backup brigade, should I need urgent assistance when David was out of town. We also wanted to express our appreciation for this urban village. In contrast to living in a trendy part of San Francisco where the turnover of residents was high, here, people raised families and lived out their lives. We met a few retired folks, two widows who had lived on the block for fifty years, an opera singer and her opera producer husband, a software engineer and his artist wife, and a few young families. Our block was home to three rabbits, two dogs, a hamster, five ducks, and an ever-multiplying number of stray cats. My parents joined the brunch, too, as did a collective of friends and family from the city—Juan Carlos, Ayi, David's parents, his brother, and a few other close friends.

After introducing myself to the new neighbors, I grabbed a slice of quiche and sat down next to Juan Carlos, curious to catch up with his life. He had graduated from his traditional Chinese medicine program and was interning at a highly regarded acupuncture clinic. His mentor was Robert (Bob) Levine, and, as it turned out, the clinic was in Berkeley, only a couple of miles away from us. I asked what Bob did, exactly.

"He takes a history, feels the pulses, then treats a patient with acupuncture and herbs." Juan Carlos's face lit up. "It's incredible to see patients heal."

"Is it gentle?"

"Yes."

"Can you give me some examples of patient cases?"

There was a patient with metastatic cancer, Juan Carlos said, who was so weak she couldn't tolerate the chemo or nausea medicines, but after starting acupuncture and herbs, she tolerated her treatments, put on weight, and had more energy. And there was a couple who struggled with infertility and had gone through all sorts of hormone shots and IVF and nothing worked, but after treating both husband and wife with herbs and acupuncture, she got pregnant naturally.

Aware that both of these cases—wasting syndromes in cancer, and infertility—were difficult to treat in the Western medicine model, I found myself thinking about another difficult case: mine.

"D'you think Bob could help my fatigue or insomnia?" I asked.

"Of course. I've seen that, too."

There were scientific studies on acupuncture's effectiveness with fatigue, chronic pain syndromes, insomnia, and mood disorders. Acupuncture, in the Western medicine terms I could understand, seemed to work by promoting the rest-and-digest phase of the autonomic nervous system, among other mechanisms. Since Chinese medicine is governed by an entirely different language and the organs are arranged in different systems, it was hard, if not impossible, to explain exactly how it worked in terms of physiology. But by this time, I needed less convincing by science. My last ER visit had opened me to the possibility of trying different paths for healing, even paths that might be considered unconventional. A Chinese-American doctor asking her Guatemalan friend about his Jewish mentor and a form of medicine two thousand years in the making that came out of her own heritage? Somehow, it all came together.

My father drove me to my first acupuncture appointment. The short distance and the small roads would have probably been manageable for me, but driving demanded so much mental energy—all the multitasking steps had to be broken down bit by bit—that I graciously accepted rides whenever they were available. He dropped me off in front of the office of Bob Levine, LAc, or licensed acupuncturist. This license meant Bob could perform acupuncture, dispense herbs, and practice other modalities within the realm of traditional Chinese medicine.

The clinic was no-frills: white walls, some magazines, a houseplant in the corner, a bottled water dispenser, and a bowl of mandarins on the end table. I filled out my patient intake forms, listening to the background music, which seemed to be Buddhist monks chanting. Then I turned my forms in, and peeled a mandarin. Oranges!

A man with white, tousled hair emerged, motioning for me to follow him. This was Bob. I introduced myself and followed his gait, which was methodical and slow, as though he were practicing tai chi with every step. In his office, the books on his shelves varied from Chinese medicine textbooks to Buddhist meditations to books written in Tibetan. When I came across Rumi's *The Big Red Book,* I liked him already.

"Is this your first time for porcu-puncture?" he said with a soft smile.

"It is," I said, laughing. I had expected a master practitioner to be very serious. "Juan Carlos referred me."

He scanned my intake form. "So, what kind of medicine do you practice?"

"Internal medicine. I'm in a small, private practice," I said. *A very small and private practice, one that no one knows about.*

"Ah, good." He winked. "Having a doctor as a patient always makes things…how shall we say…lively."

He took my right hand and rested it on a small wrist pillow, palm up, placing his fingers on my wrist. This was my radial pulse, where I would normally take a patient's heart rate. But Bob slid his fingers up and down in millimeter increments, as if he were playing the neck of a small violin. He lowered his ear toward my wrist, and raised his eyebrows.

"I'm listening to your relationship to your mother," he said, switching over to my left wrist. "Want to tell me about it?"

His question surprised me. My relationship to my mother? In my pulse? "It's pretty good—you know, like a lot of mother-daughter relationships. What do you want to know?"

"What was your relationship like during your childhood?"

This felt like a déjà vu of what I had felt with Pia—like my pulse was sending out signals for Bob to pick up, but without my consent. I felt exposed, parts of me being seen that I didn't want seen. In the thyroid doctor's office, I had felt invisible. Now I was too visible. What did I actually want?

I kept my response general. My mother and I were very different, I said, and we were from different cultures and times, and we didn't always understand each other, but we loved each other very much.

"Your body stores up experiences from a lifetime," he said. "Each organ system has its own pulse, and the stomach pulse, which often has to do with nourishment—the first forms of it, physical and emotional— often relates to a person's mother, since she's the first giver of nourishment."

As I tried to wrap my head around that, he asked me to stick out my tongue.

Then, a series of other questions.

What's your general body temperature?

Your sleep patterns?

The color and quality of your first morning urine?

The caliber of your stools?

He did the most thorough review of systems I had ever encountered, and concluded with two words: *tsa ka*.

Tsa ka is a Tibetan phrase that translates to "shock pulse." Bob explained that my body was in a state of shock, holding on to a lot of trauma, and this trauma had caused my qi, or life force energy, to stagnate. When qi is low or obstructed, disease develops. A year later, when I was strong enough to handle the news, he would tell me that my pulses—really, the organ systems they represented—were so unsynchronized during these early evaluations that, had he been blinded, he would have sworn I was three different people. That is, my life force wasn't just low, it was existentially split.

His explanation correlated with the Ecological Paradigm of Health in that multiple factors contribute to an outcome, be it negative or positive. I understood how the body didn't distinguish between emotional or mental or physical traumas (or stresses), but he was adding existential stresses into the mix, too. I thought about the distressing evangelical teachings of my childhood, and the authoritarian methods of discipline, and how they were wrapped up in my love for parents and their love for me. There was the emotional fear, yes. But I felt Bob was pointing to something closer to the intersection of body and soul.

Bob led me to another no-frills room for the treatment. There was a massage table and a shelf stocked with needles of all sizes, alcohol wipes, cotton balls, glass cups shaped like lightbulbs, and paste that resembled mud. I lay supine on the table. A heat lamp warmed my feet, and a beige curtain separated me from another patient, who was snoring. Bob wiped an area at the base of both palms with alcohol. I was nervous before he inserted the needles, and could feel myself getting warm. When I asked if it would hurt, he said the needles were already in. Done. Two needles, wispy like cat whiskers, poked out of my skin, one from each palm.

"That's it?" I said. "Um...I was kinda hoping for more."

He put his hand on my shoulder. "Trust me, this is plenty. I'm doing some releasing."

"Releasing of what?"

"Your uterus." Then he walked out and closed the door behind him.

I wondered if my uterus was contracted or inflamed, since I was pregnant when the debilitation hit. Was that what Bob meant? Western medicine had no such condition. But how did Bob know about my uterus? I had neither told him that the debilitation started with the second pregnancy, nor included that detail on my intake form. I visualized my uterus in my mind's eye: the fundus, the body, the cervical os, the fallopian tubes. But before I got too engrossed in anatomy, a tingling sensation radiated through my palms, then up my forearms, then to my armpits, and a warmth oozed throughout my torso. Within minutes, the music of chanting monks carried me into a sleep so deep that, when the intern entered and woke me, I didn't know where I was. I hadn't slept so deeply in years, even with the melatonin, magnesium, and sleep hygiene measures.

The intern removed my needles, wiped the areas with alcohol, and discharged me. I had been out for thirty minutes, but it felt like two hours. Sitting up slowly, I expected dizziness. None. No aches or inflammation-type sensations in my chest or shoulders, either. I touched my body, to make sure this was still me. The intern handed me a pouch of brown, marble-sized balls—Tibetan herbs—for me to take between treatments. I didn't know what their ingredients were, how they worked, or why I was taking them, but I was convinced of Bob's expertise and told myself to do whatever he prescribed.

I walked out with a gentle spring in my step. Slightly disoriented, but downright astonished.

At home, my mother was calling everyone to dinner. I quickly read the directions on the pouch of herbs: CRUSH FIVE BALLS, AND DRINK WITH A GLASS OF WARM WATER, TWICE A DAY. I took a whiff. They smelled like dirt. Then I crushed five and drank them down. They tasted like dirt, too—nothing I couldn't stomach, though. When I skipped to the dinner table, David looked at me like he was seeing a ghost. I talked nonstop about Bob, what he said and what he did, and how none of it made sense to my doctor's mind, but how on some deeper level, perhaps in my body, it made total sense.

My father said grace and gave particular thanks for my healing. Then we dug into my mother's beef noodle soup. The blend of flavors— garlic, soy sauce, ginger, peppercorns, scallions, and a hint of star anise—erased the taste of dirt from my mouth. Everyone was quiet, including the girls. I cleaned my bowl, and filled up on seconds. My appetite was back, too.

Cleaning up, I asked my mother why my Puo Puo chose Western medicine over traditional Chinese medicine. Puo Puo was my mother's mother, the one who had been an obstetrician-gynecologist in China and Taiwan.

"Your Puo Puo's oldest brother was a wise and powerful man," my mother said. She spoke in English, which she tried to do whenever David was around. "When Puo Puo was young, her brother told her it was important for women to get a good education, even though many women didn't go to college. When Puo Puo did well in school, he advised her to study medicine, and to choose Western medicine. It wasn't common back then, but he said it was the medicine of the future."

"He was a visionary."

My father nodded.

"I'm curious what Puo Puo thought about Chinese medicine," I pressed on.

"She thought it was like..." My mother paused to search for the correct word in English. "Like superstition."

"Like nonsense-superstition, or like cool-magic-superstition?"

"I don't know. Your Puo Puo was very rigid in some of her ideas."

So I came from a lineage of hardline rationalists, I concluded. Even in my mother's literal interpretation of the Bible—like Eve being made from Adam's rib, and Jesus feeding the crowd of five thousand with five loaves of bread and two fish—I could see that, for her, it was somehow logical. As my mother packed the leftover food away and I wiped down the table, I remembered how Bob said my stomach pulse might be connected to her. And now I found I was hungering to know who my mother was and to have her know who I was. What did she think, outside of her parents, outside of the Bible, beneath the cultural mask of *bao mienzi,* or "saving face," beyond the duties of wife and mother? And further, what did she feel?

As I went to bed, the effects of Bob's treatment were still with me. I took my magnesium and melatonin, but skipped the bath and orange goggles. David and I celebrated my body's revival. When he touched my nakedness, a few hints of sensation broke through the pervasive numbness. I can't say I was aroused organically, per se. But since my body felt stronger, I didn't feel an urge to crawl into my imaginary shoebox, which prevented me from receiving love, even as it protected me from loss. We snuggled, then transitioned naturally into sex. My symptoms were so minimal I almost didn't know what to do with myself. Afterward, I didn't notice David's nose whistling in deep slumber, because I, too, was asleep.

The peace came to an abrupt halt a little after two a.m. I was awoken by what I thought was an earthquake. I braced myself on the bed. But David was sound asleep, and the walls weren't shaking. The tremors, I realized, were inside my body. They intensified, my heart raced, and I broke into a cold sweat. I stumbled to the bathroom and opened the medicine cabinet. I still had propranolol from my hyperthyroid days (to slow my heart rate), and some valium left over from the last ER visit. I took a dose of both, wanting to avoid another ER visit at all costs.

The medicines settled the internal revolt, leaving me with a strange fluttering in my ears. *Purrrr,* I would hear every minute or so. I lay in my bed, drenched in sweat, listening to the eerie purrs until another quake shook me: a bloodcurdling cry from the other room.

Sonia was sitting up and screaming in her bed. I sat her in the glider chair with me, and tried to sing, "Hush little baby, don't you cry..." but in my drugged state, I couldn't remember the words. We rocked, and hummed, and rocked some more. Nothing soothed her. With the next "don't you cry," I began to cry, too. I was upset at both the rude take-back of my peaceable state of health, and Sonia's persistent terrors. Was she acting out because of the unpredictability of my illness? After an hour of rocking, we passed out together on the rocking chair.

When the morning birds started to chirp, Sonia and I were still in the rocking chair. I was feeling hungover, minus the headache, in a state of emotional drowsiness. David, scared of seeing me go through more withdrawal-type releases, urged me not to do any more acupuncture.

"Sure," I told David, "I'm scared of going up, then down again. But I'm more scared of staying where I am. It's clear Bob was releasing something. *Something* happening is better than nothing."

So I marched, full-steam ahead, to territories unknown.

SEVENTEEN

Two weeks after my first acupuncture session, I returned for a second. In the interim, I had continued taking the herbs twice a day, and had grown to like the earthy flavor. I had also continued the hefty doses of vitamin C, figuring extra antioxidants couldn't hurt. This time, Bob increased the number of needles to four, and inserted them in my legs and feet. These points supported my kidneys, Bob said, because I was yin-deficient. In other words, my body couldn't hold on to fluids well, which is why I was dizzy. Finally! Someone who reassured me that it wasn't my fault that I was dehydrated and dizzy—because I was drinking a ton of water!

Months later, I would learn that yin deficiency correlates in part with a dysfunction in the hormone system, resulting from any combination of the following: prolonged fight-or-flight states, endocrine-disrupting chemicals, certain nutritional deficiencies, and chronic inflammation, to name a few. The glands above the kidneys secrete various hormones, some of which influence blood pressure (hence, my dizziness) and fluid regulation (my urination). The thyroid is part of this system, too, and when one part of the system malfunctions, other parts begin to compensate. If not corrected, the whole system becomes stressed and can malfunction.

For my thyroid condition, for example, Bob wasn't merely treating the individual gland, but the entire hormone system. Then he would assess how this system affected my other systems, like the digestive system, the immune system, and the neurological system. Approaching the body in terms of systems, and not just specific target organs, could restore my body's capacity to function in a more comprehensive way.

And that's what happened. Two months into the acupuncture and herbs, I bumped up to 3.0–3.5 on the functionality scale, and it seemed to stabilize there. This marked the official end of my housebound stage. I could leave the house for short outings on most days. Though still limited, I had volleyed between 1.5–3.0 for so long that this bump felt like a hard-won climb. Stability meant reliability, reliability meant less worry, and less worry meant less time in the fight-or-flight state, which in turn meant more time in the healing state. What this translated to, in practical terms, was more flexibility. So when my parents spoke of returning to Beijing in a few weeks, I felt I could manage without them. I also encouraged them to take a short trip to visit cousins in Los Angeles in the interim. And when a couple of friends emailed about their imminent visit to the Bay Area, David and I invited them to stay for a few days.

These friends were Don and Pia. Pia was from my home state of Texas, but she and Don had recently retired to a lakeside village outside Guadalajara, Mexico. Of course, I hadn't forgotten the phone call from her, or the discoveries she had led me to. With my having more stability now, this chance to host them felt like a gift.

They arrived as though by chariot. Don's tuft of white hair was windblown, resembling feathers on a Roman helmet. Pia's silver curls shimmered against her colorful caftan. They gave hugs to the girls, then me, then David, and I introduced them to my parents. With my parents staying in the guest room, Don and Pia settled into the office, with a pull-out futon. As soon as Pia put her purse and jacket down in the office, she began to cough. I brought her a glass of water. She coughed again.

"Sorry, it's probably the dust in here," I said.

"It's not that." She looked around the room. "There's a heaviness here. In the house, actually. Do you sense it?"

I shook my head.

We joined Don and David in the living room, where she posed the same question to them. They shook their heads, too. Neither of them sensed anything off.

She asked to walk around the house. I said sure, and decided to accompany her, recalling how the house had felt depressed to me when I first saw it. When we got to the girls' room, she said the energy was heaviest in there. That made me think of Sonia's recent struggles. "You know, Sonia has been having night terrors since we moved in."

Pia was quiet for a moment. "No...well, yes. What I mean is, it's not that Sonia's distress is causing the heaviness. She senses the heaviness, and that's why she's upset."

"Sonia senses this? How can you be so sure?"

"Children detect these things much more readily than adults. Adults get too dependent on their rational minds, and lose the capacity to sense subtle energies."

I might have written that off if Pia hadn't said, "I see a tall, slender man with boxy shoulders." She waved her hand above her head in a circular motion. "His hair is thinning on top, almost bald. I think his hair is reddish-brown, maybe? It matches his plaid shirt."

The seller of our house! The two times we saw him, in fact, he was wearing plaid shirts. Shivers went down my arms.

"He was depressed," she said, "and his energy is still here."

At this point, my thoughts and feelings were all over the map. One moment I was curious, the next skeptical, then frightened. But one thing was undeniable: her visions of the seller and his energy were spot-on. My main priority was to ease Sonia's distress, so when Pia and I joined David and Don in the living room again, I was interested in exploring further. "What can we do for a toddler who's having night terrors?"

"It's simple, actually," Pia said. "Is there a Whole Foods nearby?"

I gave her the cross-streets, and Don and Pia quickly headed there in their rental car.

David looked at me. "What were you two discussing?"

I told him about the energy, Pia's vision of the seller, and the connection to Sonia's night terrors.

"You must be really desperate," he said.

"I *am* desperate. And what do we have to lose? In medicine, we're always looking for therapies that are low in risk, and high in potential gain."

Thirty minutes later, Don and Pia returned with a paper bag filled to the brim. Out came a bunch of apples, a loaf of bread, a tube of lotion, and some toothpaste. The last item they unpacked was a bundle of dried herbs. Sage, to be exact.

"This is a smudge stick," Pia explained. "They've been used in various rituals for a long time to clear up energy. What really matters, though, is the intention behind the ritual—that's what does the trick." She held up a matchstick. "May I?" I nodded, and she struck the match, lighting the edge of the bundle until smoke started to rise in thin streams. She walked from room to room, waving her arms like an orchestra conductor, asking the energy to lift. From time to time, she would breathe in the sage-scented air and exhale a drawn-out, *Ahhh.* Then she extinguished the smudge stick in the sink.

That night, Sonia slept eleven or twelve hours without a peep. I couldn't quite believe it, so I checked on her every few hours. She was always tucked under her bed covers, her round cheeks snug against her stuffed bunny, her chest gently lifting and falling, lifting and falling.

The following morning, my parents, David, and I had an early breakfast while Don and Pia slept in. Sonia was especially perky, and I commented on what a good sleeper she was. David shared with my parents all that had transpired.

David: "I wanna see if this lasts."

My father: "Maybe Sonia's finally gotten used to your new home."

My mother: "Is Pia a Christian?"

I shook my head.

"Then how do you know she's not a witch?"

My mother's caution evoked the teachings of my childhood church: *The acts of the flesh are obvious: sexual immorality, impurity, and debauchery; idolatry and witchcraft. Galatians 5:19-20.* While this stuff had spooked me for much of my life, desperation was now opening me to experiences outside the scientific method. I wasn't a total believer— perhaps what happened with Sonia was mere coincidence—but I wasn't a total skeptic either. My mind had stopped jumping to "no, it can't be" as its default response, and I was more open to whatever the Truth was, in whatever form it took. I accepted that sometimes, there would be no solid proof of the whys and the hows.

Sonia slept well the following night.

And the next.

On the last day of their visit, I sat down with Don. He was a climate scientist and physicist. I wanted to know how he understood clairvoyance to work.

"Physics can't explain these phenomena yet," he said, "but we do know that they don't operate according to the classical laws of mechanics. They're in the realm of quantum theory. Quantum theory boils down to particles and energy."

I thought back to college physics and how quantum theory had blown my rational mind, its basic principles defying logic. Like light traveling as a wave until it's observed, then traveling as a particle, as though the light particles *know* they are being watched. When Don saw me lost in thought, he added, "We don't have to make this so complicated. You know what intuition is, right?"

"Of course. The ability to perceive or express information in the form of shapes, images, and sensations, based in the right side of the brain.

"What I've learned from watching Pia all these years is that intuition is simply the act of tapping into the collective unconscious, where images and sensations arise."

As far as I understood it from my earlier readings of Carl Jung, the collective unconscious was a dimension of the human mind, containing timeless symbols and nonlinear knowledge. It was an interesting concept—but a mental construct that had nothing to do with clairvoyance, an experiential phenomenon in the realm of mysticism, metaphysics, and the paranormal. I would later learn that clairvoyance and intuition are on a spectrum—another zipper-type continuum. Someone with highly developed intuition can detect subtle energies, and when that happens, others who can't perceive the energies call them *psychic* (or, depending on their belief systems, *crazy*).

After speaking with Don about it, I searched the Internet and found multiple definitions for "intuition." The one I liked most was coined by scientists at an institute called HeartMath: "a process by which information normally outside the range of cognitive processes is sensed and perceived in the body and mind as certainty of knowledge or feeling (positive or negative) about the totality of a thing distant or yet to happen." In other words, an experiential or spatial form of knowing—like a "gut feeling," a strong hunch, a sudden image or sound, a bodily response, a dream…or, as I now thought about it, like the Japanese concept *ma,* the abstract non-form that somehow defines forms, and the in-between spaces Yeshi had spoken of. According to experiments conducted by HeartMath, women seem to access intuition more readily than men. And the heart might in fact sense subtle energies before the brain does.

When I searched under "intuition and science," significant moments in history popped up, ones I had learned about in college: Dmitri Mendeleev, the scientist who invented the periodic table of elements, and August Kekulé, a German chemist who discovered that benzene wasn't a chain, but a ring structure, which transformed the field of organic chemistry. Both of these discoveries came through revelatory dreams. The universe is a big ball of energy, Pia said, when I asked her. And everything in the universe is transferring energy around, too. I could see her point. The ears and nose and eyes and skin—and all their sensory nerves—are transducers of energy, translating energy from the outside world to information the brain can interpret. The human body is full of ions, which are, conveniently, conductors of energy. The mighty mitochondria, one type of our many cell structures, are microscopic powerhouses. And that's when Bob's words about my stagnated qi hit me: my body was a big ball of stuck energy!

I asked if Pia could lift the heaviness out of my body, just as she had for our house.

She smiled. "I can do better. I can teach you to develop your own intuition."

Silence. I preferred to be worked on and to be done with it.

"Once you learn to develop your own intuition," she said, "it will help you heal."

"I don't understand."

Pia suggested we do a visualization. I crossed my legs, straightened my back, and closed my eyes. I could hear Sonia running around in the background.

Pay attention to your breath, Pia began.

Let go of any thoughts that arise.

Breathe in, breathe out.

Five minutes or so passed.

She had me imagine I was on a tropical island. Walking through a patch of trees and brush, then coming to an open clearing, then a beach. She asked me to look left, look right, and notice any images that emerged.

Breathe in, breathe out. In, out.

I peeked at Pia. Her eyes were still closed, her lips almost smiling.

"Did you see anything?" she said, finally opening her eyes.

No. And I didn't understand the purpose of this exercise.

She told me what she saw. I appeared on the beach. I was floating above the sand in the middle of the scene. The left represented the past, and from there, a man with golden hair appeared. The right represented the future, and there was a staff planted in the sand. One of my feet was facing toward the left, the other toward the right. If I was to move to the right, I would need to hold onto the staff.

I wondered if the man with the golden hair was Kurt. If I was stuck, I must have still been holding on to him. If I was to move forward, I had to hold on to the staff. But what was the staff? And how would I let go of Kurt? I felt like I had done all I could to grieve him. Regardless of these questions, the resonance of Pia's vision convinced me to say, "I'd like to learn how to develop my intuition."

Intuition was like any art or craft: It unfolds according to each person's unique ability. Some are born with natural talents. Others, less so. But anyone can develop it, no matter their starting point. Like with music, for example. Some are blessed with perfect pitch, while others are tone-deaf, but most fall somewhere in the middle. The main thing is to practice, practice, and practice some more. Pairing intuition and reason—integrating the right and left brains—can provide more depth and breadth of knowing, just as having two eyes provides deeper and broader vision.

Later that day, in private, I tried the beach visualization. In my mind's eye, I followed Pia's guidance and envisioned myself wading through a field of greens until I came to an open beach. I waited patiently for an image to appear, but nothing emerged.

Another attempt.

Nothing.

Another.

Nothing.

After the third attempt, though, there was a distinct pressure, or a tingle, on my forehead, and a shiver ran through me.

Pia later told me that these sensations were important signals, indicating attunement, or the act of tuning deeply into myself and my environment. To tune in more deeply, she encouraged me to move into my body, even if it meant moving into my symptoms. My symptoms were so uncomfortable, I told her, and my way to endure them was to detach from them. No one, she said, could heal something she was always running away from. While I didn't remember it at the time, this was similar to something Yeshi had told me during my labor: "Don't be afraid of the pain, move *toward* it"—and indeed, when I had, the intensity of the pain lessened. All my life I had been trying to suppress my sensitivities, trying not to feel everything so intensely. And now with my health challenges, the sensitivities were heightened.

"Your intuitive nature is your healing nature is your sensitive nature," Pia said. "Your sensitivity is a gift, Cynthia."

I couldn't quite believe this could be a gift. It felt, well, *counter*intuitive. But I was intrigued by the idea of tapping into my intuition, to help identify what had caused my illness and how to continue healing. If my sensitive nature was an expression of my right brain, and my right brain might open me up to my subconscious, then all the better. Borrowing a quote from Jonas Salk, the inventor of the polio vaccine, I added to my How to Get Off the Couch list:

6. Let intuition tell your thinking mind where to look next.

EIGHTEEN

Don and Pia left the next morning, leaving me with more space to think. Where was I with my experiment? Sonia was sleeping soundly through the night again, which had restored structure to my days and allowed me to resume 2: *Reset your inner clock*. At a functionality of 3.0–3.5, I added to my circadian routine mid-afternoon gentle strolls. A block up the street was a forested park with redwoods and sturdy oaks and a songful creek. I would walk there for ten, then twelve, then fifteen minutes a day, and turn around when I reached the set of intimidating stairs along the forest's backside. The stairs—there must have been close to a hundred steps—looked like a crooked ladder that went on forever, but other park-goers told me they terminated at a high road. To me, that road could have been the North Pole. Fatigue distorted my sense of distance.

My circadian routine was now to arise from bed with the girls at six-thirty a.m., get breakfast going, then get Rosa ready for preschool. At eight a.m., David took Rosa to preschool, and I got Sonia started on *The Backyardigans* while I relaxed into my perch for visualizations. On the days I had brain fog (or "brain grog," as I started to call it), everything took longer. But I followed my schedule as closely as I could, because I never forgot the science that convinced me of the benefits of regular routines.

With regard to intuition, Pia had said the main thing was to practice, practice, and practice some more. So while no images emerged in the visualizations, I would sit and concentrate in my mind's eye. When I got bored or distracted, I would lay back against the cushions and listen to guided meditations. I still had the recordings from Yeshi. And YouTube had more meditations than I could imagine—for relaxation, anxiety, colds, and pain, even far-out ones purporting chromosomal repair, attracting wealth, and even contact with aliens. So I could have some fun with my visualizations, too.

The combination of visualizations, acupuncture, and herbs seemed to relax me. They also seemed to release more of *something*, and if I could name that something, it was my subconscious. Dreams. Memories. Reflections. Some of my dreams from this time bordered on psychedelic: strawberries marching down a sidewalk, or satyrs dancing in a water fountain in the backyard. Others were recycled childhood dreams, the two common motifs being big cats stalking me, or a tense situation causing me to want to scream, only to find I didn't have a voice. Others were streams of consciousness, or of Kurt, or dead relatives, or dead patients. They didn't startle me as they might have in the past—I figured my subconscious was trying to release any fears of death. But then, the dead people in my dreams started giving me specific messages to pass on to their living beloveds. This happened twice, within two weeks of when Don and Pia left. None of my dreams in the past were anything like these.

Frantic, I called Pia.

This was all normal, she said in a consoling voice. My consciousness was expanding, and it was important that I ground myself in my body and my surroundings. Pay attention, she said, and keep a journal of dreams and experiences, and note any correlations with events in my life. In hindsight, I might begin to see what was mere coincidence, and what felt like a "sign."

Intuition felt like the opposite of a systematized clinical trial, where variables could be controlled, at least to a certain degree. Instead of self-directed learning, intuition seemed like information that was coming to me at *its* will. The earlier paradigm shifts I had come across— getting past the *here/there* labeling of disease, the Ecological Paradigm of Health, the integrated systems approach in traditional Chinese medicine—were still in the realm of analytical reasoning, in the reality I could see and touch, paradigm shifts that trained my left brain. Intuition, on the other hand, was about training my left brain to get the hell out of the way, to be quiet, and to give my right brain a turn.

I mostly kept the more mystical occurrences private, including from David's parents and mine. His were academics and big proponents of psychotherapy who, I feared, might recommend I undergo psychoanalysis at once, if they knew. Mine were evangelicals who might recommend a special prayer meeting or an exorcism. In the meantime, if a dream took me too far away from what I knew to be sane or familiar, I would share it with David and ask him to hold me. He might have had his own reservations, but he never once judged me, and never once wavered in his support. In fact, he began to embrace what Pia had said, telling me "This is a gift. *Your* gift. Your sensitivities are giving you abilities I don't have." *He* was the staff in Pia's vision, grounding me.

As the end of my parents' stay neared, everyone seemed to grow a bit restless. Small irritations grew, minor things I did that triggered my mother, like not finishing all the food on my plate; or things my mother would do to trigger me, like pocketing for her coin collection the quarters David and I had left on the window sill for the car meters, or moving houseplants around without consulting us.

One evening, halfway through dinner, Rosa got up, went to the bathroom, and wouldn't come back. Her chicken and rice was growing cold as she danced and somersaulted in the living room. Sonia decided to join her, running off in her potty-training underwear. I laughed, trying to decide whether to intervene or let them play, but my mother, visibly irritated, brought the girls back to the dinner table.

"You must finish your dinner," she said to them. "Your mother and her sister and brothers never acted like this."

"Sure, we did," I said, still smiling at the girls.

Sternly, she shook her head. "You were well-behaved."

Now serious, I took a bite of rice. "I remember getting punished. A lot."

"You were a good baby, and a good child," my mother said. My father nodded in agreement. "Then, in high school and college, everything changed. You stopped going to church. You went to wild parties. I couldn't control you anymore."

"I wasn't all that 'good' when I was little," I said, letting out a half-laugh. "I was quiet and I followed directions, but that's because I was shy and afraid of everything."

"You were afraid? No...you were so strong-willed."

I ate my dinner, stealing glances at my parents, then staring off into space. Memory after memory surfaced, like turtles coming up for air. How I used to cover myself with band-aids, not because I had real physical wounds, but because I hurt inside. How I used to loathe team sports in P.E. class, not because it was ninety degrees in the Texas sun, but because I was always one of the last picks. How I used to skip school dances, including the prom, not because I had better things to do, but because a Chinese girl like me was invisible to the white boys.

When I emerged from my thoughts, my parents were clearing the dishes. I grabbed the sponge, wiped down the table, and went to my room. On my bed, I researched the impacts of early stresses and wondered how many of my genes were programmed in childhood and were now generating the inflammation in my shoulders or the dizziness in my head. The data on the impact of childhood stresses were well-established. Early stresses could create abnormal stress responses, favoring fight-or-flight, which generated chronic inflammation.

In addition, there was the recent discovery of epigenetics. *Epi* (above) + *genetics* (genes) is the study of gene *expression,* or the changes in how genes turn on and off. Whereas genetic mutations are rare and random occurrences that are largely out of our control, the turning on and off of genes happens daily, depending on what we eat, drink, breathe, and think. So I had a say over how some of my genes were expressed.

And there were studies of mice in which conditioned responses to trauma in one generation created epigenetic patterns that passed down to one, even two, generations. In human studies, one study showed a higher incidence of mood disorders in children born to mothers who lived through a famine; in another, heavier sons were born to fathers who smoked before puberty, and both of these studies found associated epigenetic evidence. One ambitious study concluded that epigenetic patterns in the children of Holocaust survivors correlated with vulnerability to stress. My parents and grandparents, then, might have had input into the expression of my genes, too.

The day before my parents left, I was sitting in my perch, watching them pack and clean. What were *their* stresses? I wondered. And their parents' stresses? What epigenetic patterns did each generation inherit, and what did the generations before them inherit, and so on? Applying this information to the Ecological Paradigm of Health and the Chinese medicine systems model, I wondered, could their stress loads have contributed to my cumulative stresses? Did some of my fatigue and dizziness not even begin with me? And what about the thyroid conditions of my father, sister, and younger brother—did they also derive in part from earlier generations?

The lore from my mother's lineage was more complete, so I closed my eyes and lay back in my perch, picturing in my mind's eye my mother, who was rail-thin during high school and college because she was studying so hard she didn't have time to eat; upon getting married, at age twenty-three, she weighed less than ninety pounds. And her mother, my Puo Puo, who fled from city to city during China's war with Japan, each of her five children born in a different city; and who, while raising and protecting them, was also managing her profession as a doctor. And Puo Puo's mother, my great-grandmother, who as a young girl was both a cook for the family and a servant to her mother's every wish, brushing and pinning her mother's hair into a bun, and washing her feet before bed. And all the way back to the earliest known ancestor on my mother's side, a revolutionary poet named Luo Binwang in the Tang Dynasty, who stood up against the tyranny of a ruthless empress. As their descendant, I would never know what patterns of stress I had received. All I could do was consider the potential of inherited stresses—and it felt like a radioactive tracer with a half-life that spanned not hours or days, but multiple generations.

I was interested in these questions, not to assign blame, but to understand. I fantasized about having a conversation with my parents, an exchange of mutual compassion in which we acknowledged everyone's unique sufferings, emotional and mental and physical. If intention could clear the heaviness in a house, I wondered if it might also clear the heaviness in my genes—a few *click-click-clicks* of the epigenetic switches, and maybe the genes that coded for inflammation might turn off. If I could learn to do this for myself, I might hope to teach the same to my girls.

A probe into the past wasn't without risks. There were deep cultural rules embedded within our family, and digging up past traumas could be seen as disrespectful, ungrateful, selfish, or just plain painful. The last thing I wanted to do was to cause my parents grief. They had flown halfway around the world at the drop of a hat, demonstrating their love through cooking, chauffeuring, unpacking boxes, and sweeping away balls of dust. My heart raced all morning and afternoon. When David came back from work, I told him the conversation I hoped for, and asked if I was selfish or disrespectful for wanting it.

"No," he said, looking into my eyes.

"No?" I asked.

"No," he repeated.

I must have asked him to repeat it to me a hundred times.

After dinner, I knew it was now or never. They were due to fly back to Beijing the next day. My mother was sitting in the nook of the bay windows, opposite my perch. It was unusual for her not to be engaged with some kind of busyness, even if just picking dead leaves off the houseplants. She almost felt *too* available, and I wondered if I was emitting some sort of signal she was unconsciously picking up. I made us two cups of tea and sat down. We started talking about ordinary things, like the local Chinese church they had visited the past Sunday, and the logistics of their return home. So it surprised me when she asked out of the blue, "Is this still your thyroid?" in a mixture of Mandarin and English.

"Yes," I said, knowing *this* referred to my health. I wasn't sure how much else to say.

"Why don't you find a doctor who can give you the right cure?"

"It's more complicated than that...how can I make it simple? My nerves, hormones, and immune system aren't working right, so my balance is off. Like right now, I feel like I'm on a boat, even though we're just sitting here talking...and sometimes my muscles and joints feel like I just ran a marathon...and I feel like I've had the flu for three years now."

The expression on her face became anguished. I felt like I had said too much, but from my perspective, I had hardly said anything at all.

"I don't understand," she said.

"I don't really either."

Swirls of steam rose from my cup.

"So, Mom." I cleared my throat. "I've been researching autoimmune diseases—that's what I have, a condition where my body is attacking itself...and I've been thinking about my childhood...a lot of these kinds of conditions can be traced back to early childhood."

She looked toward me, but not into my eyes. I wondered what I would say next, how to phrase it, but my mother steered the conversation forward. "You said when you were little, you were scared all the time. I find that hard to believe."

I nodded gently.

"What about all those trips to Disney World and the national parks, the designer clothes we didn't have the money for, but we bought for you anyway—how come all you remember is the bad stuff?"

"I remember the good times, too. But they don't feel as large as the harder times. I remember getting punished a lot, and being told *Gai si*, You should die, and just feeling lost. I wanted you to be proud of me. I knew I wasn't the smartest kid, but when I told you I was thinking of medical school, you and Dad didn't think I had what it took."

"We weren't proud of you?" Her voice tensed up. "Is that what you thought?"

"I'm sorry. I'm not blaming you. I'm just trying to have my experience acknowledged."

My mother's lips quivered. "I grew up watching my own mother work so hard as a doctor. Her patients always came first, and her health suffered. She had stomach problems, and she lost a lot of weight. Even after she retired, she couldn't enjoy life because she was constantly worried about germs. I didn't want the same to happen to you, as a doctor. Your father and I came to this country to give the four of you a better life. You've had freedoms we never had. You've had too much freedom. You even have freedom to talk to me like this, which I never had."

I sat back, saddened—both that I had misinterpreted her ambivalence in my pursuit of medicine as a lack of faith in me, and that she was avoiding the essence of what I was saying.

"I misunderstood," I said. "I'm sorry."

We sipped our tea in silence for a few minutes.

Glad she didn't get up and leave, I tried to shift the focus. "How was I as a baby and a toddler?"

My mother stared out the window, as if looking into an imaginary scrapbook. "When you were born, I was two weeks past my due date. Other than having to be induced, you were a very healthy baby, almost eight pounds." Then her voice began to crack. "At three weeks old, you got a cough that wouldn't go away. The doctors gave you seven days of antibiotics, and it got better. But a month later, you got sick again, a cough, plus an ear infection. You were on antibiotics for fourteen days! During your first year, in total, you took four rounds of antibiotics." Her eyes welled up and her nose reddened at its tip.

"Okay, so I got sick a lot," I said, trying to lighten things up. "Rosa and Sonia get colds all the time. That's common for babies and kids."

"If you remember, your Nai Nai"—my father's mother—"was a smoker. She smoked a pack a day, then quit when you were in high school. Since your sister was only fifteen months old when you were born, Nai Nai lived with us for six months to help. She used to chew table food into mash before feeding it to you. That's how the Chinese used to do it."

I wasn't sure why she was telling me this, but I could sense her mounting discomfort.

"After the second time you got sick," she continued, "I figured you were sensitive to her smoking and that's why you were getting sick. But

I didn't stand up to her. I didn't feel I could. She was my mother-in-law. And now, you're sick. You've suffered so much. To learn you were scared as a child when I disciplined you... *Gai si*—it was just a phrase like 'damn it,' it wasn't directed at you... I don't remember you feeling bad about yourself... I really don't remember a lot, but if I did anything to make you feel bad, I'm sorry." Her body trembled as she broke down.

"It's not your fault, Mom." I wanted to hug her, but didn't know how, exactly. She had said so much, all jumbled together, leaving me in a state of shock. Having wanted for so long to heal the divide between us, to have open and direct exchanges without any shame—and now, finally having one—I didn't know how to relate to her. My face probably looked wooden, the way it had in early photos. There was perhaps a deeper divide, too, which I wouldn't appreciate until much later. A divide not between her and me, but within my own self. I couldn't fully access my own grief.

I continued to watch her body shake, witnessing in her outpour something clearer than words could ever convey—a lifetime's worth of her self-sacrifice to family and elders. Over several minutes, I tried to *see* her. Not as my mother, but as a woman who perhaps had never felt seen either. Hers was a different kind of courage.

When she collected herself and got up to tidy up the kitchen, I reached over, put my hand on her shoulder, and could have sworn I felt some switches go off—*click-click-click*—deep within my cells.

7. Change your thoughts, change your genes.

NINETEEN

My parents left for Beijing the next day. Before their departure, I didn't care about being reserved in my gratitude for them. Many times over, I said *Xie xie,* thanking them, and hugged them, and said "I love you." My mother looked me in the eyes, and they both hugged me long and hard. "We will continue to pray for you," my father said, which I now understood to be their greatest gesture of love.

Cleaning out the guest room, I recounted all that had happened during their three-month stay, most of which couldn't have happened without their support: we settled into a new home in a new city; I started acupuncture and herbs, and began learning an integrated approach to healing the systems of the body; I opened to the power of intuition; I dug into epigenetics and the potential to change gene expression; and I ventured into some difficult but healing talks with my parents. This steep and brisk learning curve rivaled that of medical school.

With my parents gone, David and I had to readjust to the workload of childcare and chores. His workweeks continued to be full, so in addition to being the primary parent during the week, I saw my other role as being his primary support person, enabling his work for the sustainability of the planet. David was now highly sought after as a consultant, policy adviser, and speaker. He gave presentations, often keynotes, and collaborated with celebrities such as Daryl Hannah, Robert Redford, and Bonnie Raitt. Once, he did a roundtable on electric vehicles with Arnold Schwarzenegger (who was, incidentally, working on another *Terminator* sequel). For his trailblazing work, David received many awards.

On the weekends, when David was home, the imbalances in domestic duties didn't melt away simply because we were finding ways to love each other better. Dishes, laundry, and dust still created tension. I began to notice, however, that the heat they created, at least within myself, was cooler. If I had to raise my voice to get him to help clean up after dinner, loading the dishes and wiping down the table were all that was about. Having addressed some of my formative wounds with my parents seemed to reduce the stakes with David—just as the marriage counselor had said it would. One night, when I first recognized this, amid my irritation with him, I remarked, "Oh, my God, it's *only* about the dishes!" He didn't seem to understand, so I said it again. "It's *only* about the dishes!"

I didn't take these revelations for granted. I also didn't overlook my slow-growing freedom in the big world, directly related to my ability to drive. I still avoided freeways, but I could reliably go to the grocery store, the preschool, and Bob's clinic. Chronic fatigue whittles down the busyness of life to the absolute necessities. As long as I could be mentally present, the smallest blessings of ordinary life felt grand.

My visits to Bob were now spaced out to once a month. Although he was still releasing traumas and balancing the hormone and nervous systems, he changed his primary focus to boosting my qi; my life force, in addition to being obstructed, was deficient. Boosting qi was a longer-term issue than releasing obstructions. Just as it's faster to open up a dam to get water flowing again than it is to wait for a reservoir to fill up after being close to empty, the prognosis on boosting qi was months, not weeks. Sometimes, years.

"I know healing happens at its own pace," I said, "but is there any way we can make it go faster?"

"Qigong," Bob said.

He was suggesting that a mind-body practice could boost my body's energy naturally. I had seen people doing it in the public squares when I had visited my parents in Beijing. There was also a small group in Dolores Park that I had noticed when we lived there. Later, I would learn that qigong, a moving meditation, was the foundation of traditional Chinese medicine, was applied in Confucianism to improve moral character, and was used in martial arts to improve forms and strategies.

"I'll do a treatment right now to boost your qi," Bob said, "but qigong can supplement acupuncture in the long term."

Unconvinced, I lay supine on the table. He inserted the needles, upwards of ten or twelve now, because my internal systems could handle more. A few in the ears, others scattered on the arms and legs, and one on the crown of the head, poking out like a radio antenna. He left the room, and I drifted off again, into a fully relaxed state, listening to the chants of Buddhist monks playing in the background.

Each treatment resulted in a temporary surge of energy, but the effects were hard to sustain between the treatments, even with the herbs. Bob taught me to give myself acupuncture on four points, for general well-being and autonomic nervous system support. David likened me to a plug-in hybrid, with Bob's needles to charge me up on a monthly basis. But what I needed more of was energy efficiency, he said, so as not to waste the energy coming in, and I also needed a better way to store the energy.

Connecting David's analogy to what I knew about energy generation in the body, I looked up mitochondria and inflammation. Mitochondria are the powerhouses of the cell, averaging a thousand per cell. Energy production in the body declines by two primary means: (1) a reduction in the total number of mitochondria, or (2) an impairment in existing mitochondria. For the former, aging and lack of exercise are the two main causes. For the latter, I discovered, the main causes are toxicities, nutrient deficiencies—and inflammation! Exercise, it turned out, can increase the number *and* function of mitochondria—but this required strength and stamina I didn't think I had. And toxicities and nutrients felt like black holes I wasn't yet ready to explore. As for the inflammation, I was already doing my best to reduce it. How would I get out of this conundrum?

The answer came in a circuitous way. One of our neighbors had adopted kittens. Rosa and Sonia had only seen cats a handful of times, because David was allergic to their dander. On a day when I had a little more energy, I took the girls over, where two gray balls of fur were nestled into our neighbor's couch. Rosa held one, and Sonia the other. The kittens purred. The girls giggled. Sonia dangled some red yarn from her fingers, and the kittens leapt to and fro. Rosa fed them some kibble. After a thirty-minute lovefest, I had to pry their arms open to return the kittens to the owner.

When we got home, Sonia sneezed. Again. And again. Within minutes, her eyes turned pink, puffy, and itchy. Resurrecting my pen-light and stethoscope, I checked her mouth for swelling, her lungs for wheezing. Clear on both fronts. David walked in as I was holding a cool washcloth to her head and giving her some Benadryl.

"You can't hold kitties anymore," Rosa explained.

Sonia frowned. "Kitty," she said several times.

"She's allergic to cats, too," I said, looking at David.

"Ah, poor girl," he said. "If only you could snap your fingers and make it go away. Like that patient you told me about."

David was referring to a patient I had observed during my psychia-try rotation. A young man in his thirties, having a timid demeanor and wearing sunglasses indoors, he had dissociative identity disorder, once called "multiple personality disorder." I was rounding with his long-time psychoanalyst, who explained that this patient had five or six distinct personas, each one unaware of what the others experienced.

The analyst began with the first persona, whom I'll call Johnny. He pulled out a Ziplock baggie with a few strands of cat hair. Johnny was extremely allergic to cats. Within a minute or so, his lungs wheezed and his skin flared into hives, and he began to panic. Instead of administer-ing an inhaler or antihistamines, the therapist told Johnny, "I'll count backward from ten to one, and at the snap of my fingers, I want [Martin] to take over. Ten, nine, eight...two, one." *Snap!*

Johnny switched into Martin. The wheezing and rashes resolved in an instant, as though the patient had received a shot of high-dose ste-roids. I couldn't explain it then, so I deemed Johnny to be somaticizing, or converting some emotional symptom he was experiencing into physi-cal ones. In other words, I had judged him as many people judged those with chronic fatigue, or any syndrome we can't readily explain.

Now, as I sat in my perch, my eyes opened to a hidden perspective. I understood that changing thoughts could change genes, but somehow I had only conceived of this happening *in the brain*. I hadn't quite realized the extent of the changes possible *in the body*. If Johnny's alternate personas could dramatically alter his body's inflammatory responses, could others without dissociative identity disorder, like me, do the same?

Later that week, I took the girls to the public library. They picked out *George and Martha*, *Jam for Frances*, and picture books of animals in the wild. I picked out a book called *The Brain That Changes Itself*, by a Canadian psychiatrist, Dr. Norman Doidge. Dr. Doidge profiled patients who had recovered from profound illnesses through targeted brain exercises. This was the then-new concept of neuroplasticity, the ability of neurons—the spiderlike cells in the nervous system, numbering a hundred billion in a single person, that transmit impulses to organs and muscles—to rewire their connections. While the neurons themselves are fixed, they can change how they connect. They can form different weblike patterns, some that promote inflammation (as in Johnny), and others that reduce inflammation (as in Martin).

As Doidge described it, neuroplasticity built upon what I had learned so far about detoxification, environmental health, and epigenetics. Detoxification addressed changes on an organ level. Environmental health addressed changes on a community level. Epigenetics addressed changes on the gene level. And now, neuroplasticity was addressing changes on the systems level.

Like Bob's acupuncture treatments, neuroplasticity supports the nervous system as a whole, and since the nervous system connects with other systems, like the hormone and immune systems, the impacts can be widespread, potentially synergizing with other healing interventions. And like Pia had said, we can't heal something we're always running away from. Neuroplasticity was saying the same thing, that healing the body requires that we *inhabit* the body. It seemed I needed more than short walks to the park to bring any potentially positive brain changes down into my body; perhaps the detachment I had long used as my coping skill had left my brain and body unable to reconnect.

It turned out there was a low-tech, low-cost, easily accessible means to achieve this: mind-body practices. For example, the qigong Bob had referenced earlier. Now bolstered by science, this recommendation moved in my mind from the "interesting, I'll think about it" list to the "valid, must check it out" list. I searched for local qigong studios and there were several in my area. But I got held up, waiting for a day when I felt motivated enough to arrange for childcare, do all my self-care measures, and drive myself over.

Six months passed.

Then I received an email from Yeshi the midwife. I hadn't heard from her in a couple of years, but we had been sending her cards during the winter holidays, along with photos of the girls. In her email, she wrote that she had retired from midwifery. Her new venture was facilitating workshops for mothers and grandmothers, and she was reaching out to former clients like me. I was so glad to hear from her, agreed to circulate information about her work, and added a brief update about our family's move to Berkeley. She replied that she came regularly to Berkeley to babysit her granddaughter. We arranged to meet for lunch.

We met at a café. Yeshi had cut her hair so her silver curls were no longer in a bun, but light and buoyant against her face. Wearing a necklace of abalone shell and large hoop earrings, she looked particularly vibrant.

"I want some of what *you're* having," I said.

"You want to know my secret for the past two years?" she said. "Qigong."

I nearly choked on my tea.

"I've been in a teacher training program with my teacher, Master Gu. He's holding a daylong workshop in a couple of weeks. If you're interested, I'd love for you to join me."

Had life always been so serendipitous, or was this timing sheer coincidence? I wasn't sure, but I was paying attention now.

Two weeks later, David dropped me off at a meditation center while he and the girls met up with his cousins. I had taken my herbs and stayed especially close to my circadian routine, to maximize my chances of attending the workshop. Yeshi was sitting front-row, center, in an auditorium of a hundred and fifty or so people. She briefly introduced me to Master Gu, then showed me to the seat she had saved next to her.

I watched as Master Gu sat in a quiet, preparatory meditation. His build was slender and his head shaved, and he wore wire-rim glasses and a yellow satin tang suit, loose with button knots and a Mandarin collar. I had read Master Gu's personal story online prior to the workshop. It was filled with extraordinary hardships, from enduring China's Cultural Revolution to chronic health challenges that led him to qigong. But as he finished his meditation and stood in front of us, ready to begin the class, there was no trace whatsoever of these hardships. The smile across his face seemed genuine; his laughter reverberated throughout the room.

He started us off with a sitting meditation, having us envision qi as a field of energy in all directions, expanding out to the horizon. Qi wasn't just in us, he said, it was everywhere, flowing in and out of us like air. Then he had us envision the same qi field flowing up through our feet, all the way through our bodies to the crown of our heads, then flowing up to the heavens. After five minutes, he asked us to stand up. It was time to work the qi. "Stand up tall," he said. "Tuck your tailbone in and hold your shoulders back, chin tucked slightly under. This is the posture of health." After all my years of slouching, of holding myself smaller to conform to other people's ideas of how a Chinese woman ought to look, I stood taller than ever before.

The practice was called "Lift Qi Up, Pour Qi Down," and the movements were exactly as the name suggests. The palms and arms held a ball of energy, and the slow, intentional, back-and-forth motions had us kneading the ball in rhythmic strokes. We raised our arms up, then down, and we brought our fingertips to resting positions along various meridians, the same points used for acupuncture. All these movements were an effort to keep the qi flowing through our bodies and to remove any obstructions.

Halfway through the practice, I was holding my arms in a circle above my head for I don't know how long. My muscles ached with the sheer weight of my arms, then began to shake.

"Feel the intensity," Master Gu said.

My shoulders emitted a sharp pain where they connected to the arm bone.

"Notice where you feel the intensity," Master Gu continued. "This is 'aliveness,'" he said, laughing heartily. "You're alive! Let go of the labels of good and bad… Just observe and feel your body as pure energy."

Finally, Master Gu coached us to bring down our arms, slowly… slowly…harnessing the qi and bringing it into our navel. As I rested my hands in my *dantian,* or energy center, a shiver ran through my body, head to toe. *Ahhhh.*

By the end of the thirty-minute practice, I was spent. My feet had been planted in the same place, they hadn't moved an inch, and we had worked only with the weight of our limbs. Still, I needed a rest. And it wasn't just me. Other beginners around me needed a rest, too. I decided I couldn't just sit it out; I needed to lie down at home. So at the next break, only an hour into the six-hour day, I thanked Yeshi and Master Gu.

"The key to building your qi is repetition," he said. "Practice daily, twice a day if possible. Even if it's just five minutes." The entire practice, among others, was on his website, so I could practice at home.

"When's the ideal time?" I asked, wanting to build this into my circadian routine.

"It's good to get the qi flowing in the morning."

"Mornings are generally slow for me, energy-wise."

"Then you can sit and visualize the practice, which is healing, too."

I called David and asked him to pick me up whenever he and the girls were done hanging out with the cousins. During the wait, I started putting together the ill-matched puzzle pieces of my journey thus far, and realized they weren't so ill-matched after all. Visualizing the practice if I couldn't practice it—that was the principle of neuroplasticity. The shiver I felt at the end of the practice—that was what Pia called attunement, or tuning into the field of the collective unconscious. In physiological terms, the shiver represented the activation of the rest-and-digest state. Mind-body practices like qigong brought them all together.

David scooped me up. On the drive home, the girls fell asleep in their car seats. I reclined my seat, feeling sore and dizzy, like I was coming down with the flu again. But instead of labeling this as bad, as Master Gu had encouraged us to resist doing, I imagined qi trying to flow and the mitochondria in my muscles multiplying from the mind-body practices I had just done. Instead of getting down on myself for overdoing it, I was pleased with myself for having shown up and partici-pated. It was crazy, but that one simple shift—removing the label of "bad"—seemed to mitigate the reaction some.

At home, I sat down with my daily schedule and wrote in *qigong* after breakfast, which I could do along with my visualizations, and also before bed. I committed to starting that very night. So after eating dinner, getting the girls washed and tucked in, putting on my orange goggles, and taking my magnesium and melatonin, I logged onto the Chi Center website. Still spent from the day, I scanned the list of prac-tices and clicked on "Sound Healing." *Just five minutes,* I told myself.

Master Gu's video was an introduction to fifteen different sounds. Chanted aloud, these sounds generate unique vibrations for the five different organ systems and connect them to the mind. Each organ has a physical function as well as an emotional one. For example, a stagnant heart harbors jealousy, but an open one expresses joy and connection; a stagnant lung churns grief, but an open one releases compassion. Long before the science on neuroplasticity, this ancient system had already understood that the distinction between mental, physical, and emotional health was in concept only.

I recited along with the recording:

Xin... xian... xing...
Eh... eu... ying...
Gang... foo... zhong...
Tu... jiu... ling...
Sang... si... song...

David entered the bedroom during the *tu-tu-tu!* sound and laughed so loudly I thought he would awaken the girls at the other end of the hall.

"Sounds like you're spitting at someone you truly despise," he said.

"That's the sound for the liver, which transforms anger."

I felt a deep satisfaction, akin to hitting a punching bag. Was this how my ancestors released their grief? I wondered, as I climbed into bed.

My sleep wasn't any better that night. Per usual, I got two hours here, two hours there. But when morning arrived, I realized, Wait a minute, I didn't have to pee, not once all night! And after only the very first day of qigong! I could only assume the practice brought the rest-and-digest state from my mind down into my body. With my body no longer cranking out stress hormones, perhaps my glands had shifted toward making more fluid-regulating hormones, ones that signaled to my kidneys to better hold on to salt and fluids.

I couldn't believe it, I had to believe it.

To mark the continued success of my How to Get Off the Couch experiment, I went to the video store one night and picked out a few movies for David and me.

"Reese?" he said.

I shook my head.

"Woody?"

I shook my head and held up the original *Star Wars* trilogy.

David's jaw dropped. "You can handle this?"

I nodded and gave a little smile. "I wanna watch it again, now that I finally have a sense of what the Force is. Yoda was a qigong master!"

The Force was all around me and within me. Waiting to be harnessed.

8. Inhabit your body.

TWENTY

2010

Several months passed.

Every morning, I did the Lift Qi Up, Pour Qi Down practice from the workshop, and came to memorize the sequence of movements. Sometimes I incorporated the sound healing, too. By doing this in the park up the block, I consolidated 4: *Get a daily dose of nature* and 8: *Inhabit your body.* My body became more limber. The shivers increased, bringing me more easily into attunement and making my visualizations more vivid. The green hummingbird often appeared in the beach of my mind's eye, reassuring me of an impending renewal.

It wasn't all bright. Other times, there were rats running around my visualizations, taking over the beach and gnawing on carcasses littered throughout. I was horrified at first, then I came to understand how these light and dark images fit into the Newtonian law of balanced forces. As much as I feared the dark, the light could only *be* if there was dark.

My health changed in unexpected ways. The frequent urination was only the first in the string of "accessory symptoms" to diminish or resolve. The aches and pains in my shoulders and chest soon decreased, the heart palpitations became less frequent, and the windedness in my chest essentially disappeared. I stopped needing to drink salty water on a daily basis. And my sleep, though still a challenge, became less erratic. I took these improvements to reflect less underlying inflammation, and with less inflammation, my mitochondrial powerhouses could produce more energy. I was capable of a few hours of light housework and computer work every day, and also daily errands and short outings. My walks increased to thirty minutes, three or four days a week. Knowing the poor prognosis on recovering from chronic fatigue, I was excited to be beating the odds. On the functionality scale, I was now at 4–4.5.

The 4–4.5 was a new set point, but there was still a lot of up and down. A stable set point didn't necessarily mean no variations, day to day or week to week. It meant that, if there was a setback, I would more easily bounce back to the new set point. In some ways, it felt like time stood still, the same week playing over and over again. In other ways, however, time moved swiftly. Sonia started preschool. Rosa started kindergarten. David's parents moved from San Francisco to Berkeley. And we hired Dolma, a young and able Tibetan woman, to help out a few afternoons a week.

At one point, mired in day-to-day stuff and feeling I had lost sight of my general direction on the corkscrew path of healing, I asked David what he thought about a getaway.

"You're ready for a trip?" He had a pep in his voice I had forgotten.

"A *small* trip."

"Want to come on my business trip to Hawaii?"

Hawaii felt as distant as the moon. "I was thinking more like Point Reyes."

So it was in the sanctuary of the Point Reyes National Seashore, an hour away on the Northern California coast, that I turned forty. I received emails, calls, and text messages wishing me well, and the *Oh, lordy, look who's forty* kinds of comments. But a new decade didn't feel like a big deal to me. The bigger deal was the glorious big world in front of my eyes, and there was no better place to 4: *Get a daily dose of nature.*

It was sunny and temperate along the coast that weekend. The tufted grasses were turning yellow in the autumn sun, and the live oaks had dropped most of their leaves. Autumn was my favorite season and dusk my favorite time of day. Close to dusk, David and I took the girls on a gentle, thirty-minute walk along a narrow inlet, where we saw elk and ground squirrels and dozens of species of birds. When the trail got too narrow and the sea a thousand feet below was undulating and I began to lose my equilibrium, I grabbed hold of David's arm—my staff—and carefully turned around.

Walking the outer edges of the earth, if only for a moment, I received the greatest gift, one I couldn't have asked for because I didn't know it was possible: I forgot my identity as a patient. I was simply part of an *n* of thousands of hikers to have graced these cliffs.

The glow of the seashore carried over to Berkeley, for a few days anyhow. Then the urban rhythms took over. David left for a trip to the East Coast. The girls were back in school. And the following week, Rosa had a dentist appointment—her first. She went to kindergarten that day, and after resting and having Dolma pick her up from school, I had the energy to take her to the appointment.

Rosa was a decent brusher, a good eater, and she didn't eat too many sweets. So while the hygienist cleaned Rosa's teeth, I waited at ease, flipping through *Good Housekeeping*. When the hygienist finished, the dentist examined Rosa and called me over.

"Your daughter has some cavities," she said, looking up.

"Some?" I said. "You mean, more than one?"

"Six, to be exact."

"Six?!"

"Don't blame yourself, it's probably genetic."

I had heard that before, with my thyroiditis. Part of me wished to just patch up her cavities, chalk it up to genes, and be done with it. But the knowledge I had now told me that if we didn't identify and address underlying factors, she might be at an increased risk for developing other health issues, and given that autoimmunity ran in our family… *Ugh*, the health and illness zipper-type continuum suddenly felt infinite. There would always be something we could do to zip it *here*-ward. Could a mother-doctor's work ever be done?

At home, I sat in meditation, first releasing my anger with several rounds of *tu-tu-tu!* sound healing chants. More relaxed, I felt a pressure in my forehead, a shiver down my shoulders. An intuitive signal? I wondered. I went back into meditation and saw in my mind's eye a beautiful, grassy field, golden out to the horizon. It resembled the trail we had hiked in Point Reyes. What did this mean—more time in nature? Whom did it apply to, Rosa or me? Or was it just a random blip in my consciousness? Either way, the vision was so relaxing that I held it for several minutes. Then I went to my laptop for more concrete answers.

My initial search for cavities in children came up with the usual poor hygiene stuff—not brushing enough, drinking sodas and juice, and so forth. Digging deeper, I came across the work of Dr. Weston A. Price. Dr. Price was a dentist who practiced during the early- to mid-1900s. He noted cavity rates in children exploding before his eyes. As this was the era of industrialization, he wondered if this trend was caused by a sudden increase in processed foods. To investigate, he traveled the world, visiting indigenous tribes who were still eating their cultural diets. He examined their teeth, took photographs, and observed their food and lifestyle habits. What he found, even in cultures with minimal hygiene practices, were cavity-free mouths and strong, symmetrical facial bones. Their jaws were wide, their cheeks high. There was no need, then, for extractions or orthodontia.

Food isn't just generic energy—it's molecular information. In addition to fueling the mitochondrial powerhouses, food tells our cells what to do and serves as building blocks for hormones, brain chemicals, and cell membranes. Because the human body is constantly turning over—cells die and new cells are constantly forming—we need a steady supply of these building materials to keep the body running smoothly. Processed foods carry with them rancid vegetable oils, high amounts of sugar, other refined starches, and artificial flavors and colors. Rancid oils can damage nerves and blood vessels. High fructose corn syrup can cause weight gain and increase inflammation, as well as increase cancer risks. Artificial food coloring can cause allergies, as well as hyperactivity and irritability. These modern modified foods seemed as harmful as the toxic chemicals I had researched earlier.

Traditional foods, on the other hand, were foods the human body had evolved with over millions of years. Whether the diets were high-meat, high-fat, vegetarian, or seafood, they shared some core features: fermented foods, bone broths and hearty stews (and, if meat was used, the whole animal, including organ meats), a large assortment of vegetables, fruits, seeds, and nuts. Our teeth, Price argued, aren't simply tools for biting and chewing. Along with hair and skin, they are signposts for overall health, and diseased teeth are signposts for underlying inflammation. So while medicines and cutting-edge procedures might treat cavities or gum disease after the fact, cooking and eating real foods could heal and prevent them.

Why had I not learned any of this in medical school? The standard curriculum required only a few days of nutrition in the entire four years. And my nutrition classes focused on extreme deficiencies and excesses, cases that usually warrant hospitalization, not the more common undernourished (and overfed) typical American. In fact, I couldn't recall the word "food" ever being referenced. Nursing stations were stocked with graham crackers and chocolate bars. Noontime conferences served Chinese fast food, pizza, and on occasion, subway sandwiches. On call nights, we often ate at McDonald's, which was on the first floor of the hospital, next to the main elevators. All the times I stood in line for French fries and a patient stood in the next line over, wearing his hospital gown and toting his urine bag, and then a few hours later becoming "volume overloaded" and needing me to prescribe an IV medication to remove excess salt and fluid from his body—it was so much the norm, I couldn't see the irony.

I sat facing my laptop, realizing I had to make up for lost time and learn about nutrient-dense cooking. Never having had my mother's talent in the kitchen, I cooked to feed my family, but not necessarily to nourish them. So I began to scour websites for easy recipes. My eyes glazed over at the number and assortment of dishes. Days into this tedium, a neighbor, one of the duck keepers, stopped by to give us some of her fresh eggs. They were larger than chicken eggs, the shells more delicate, with a slightly bluish hue. Excited, I told her about Dr. Price and my recent learnings, and at the end of our brief conversation, she mentioned Three Stone Hearth. This was a kitchen co-op a mile from our house that prepared food the ancestral way, à la Dr. Price, and hosted classes on bone broth and fermentation.

The following Saturday, with David gone on another trip, I brought the girls to a how-to workshop on bone broth. Three Stone Hearth was a warehouse space with a small retail food pantry in front, various work spaces in the middle, and a large commercial kitchen along the back. The shelves were stocked with glass milk bottles, recyclable mason jars, and empty egg cartons. Rosa and Sonia headed straight for the small play area, made up of a miniature barn, a rocking horse, and an assortment of wooden blocks.

While they played, the broth class started. There were ten or so of us, a mix of men and women, decked out with aprons and disposable gloves. The instructor rolled out a cart of beef bones and browned meat, and threw them in an industrial-size stockpot, then added filtered water and some apple cider vinegar. "Forty-eight hours," he said.

"Wait, that's it?" I said. "Two ingredients, plus water, and simmer for two days?"

"Yup," he said.

Even *I* could do this. Astonished at having taken a class for something so simple, I later found out it wasn't really a class, but the introductory portion of the "broth bar," a happy hour for ancestral foodies. As we gathered around a table for broth fresh off the stove, the instructor raised his mug and cheered, "Here's to the gut!"

Sipping the golden elixir, I asked the instructor why the gut was such a big deal. He spoke of the microbiome and how paramount it was to good health. The microbiome, or flora, is the community of bacteria, viruses, yeasts, and parasites that live in our guts, mouths, airways, genitals, and skin. In the gut, they help to digest food, maintain the integrity of the gut lining, and metabolize hormones, among other functions. A person's gut flora is seeded before birth by the mother's flora, and continues to evolve into an adult-like flora until five years of age. These microorganisms are the keepers of the peace, and they outnumber the body's cells ten to one. In other words, I was more *E. coli* and *Lactobacillus* than I was human.

I would later research this information myself. He wasn't exaggerating the gut's importance to health. The gut flora is, in fact, a microecosystem. As such, the flora can be altered by external influences that make the ecosystem either vulnerable or resilient. Factors that increase vulnerability can be classified into those that reduce the *diversity* of flora (like frequent antibiotic use, or a "monoculture" diet of refined, nutrient- and fiber-poor foods) or those that change the *composition* of the gut flora (like chronic fight-or-flight states, infections, or toxic chemicals). Factors that increase resilience are the opposite (foods rich in plant fiber, a diversity of nutrients, and being in a largely rest-and-digest state). At a certain threshold of stresses, the gut can generate inflammation; unchecked inflammation can break down the gut lining, which can spread the inflammation into the body. This matters in autoimmune diseases because the gut flora is a key "trainer" of the immune system, helping to teach what is a foreign invader that doesn't belong in the body, and what is, in fact, part of one's total "self." It made sense, then, that a lot of patients with mystery illnesses or chronic fatigue have imbalanced flora.

As the broth bar concluded, my doctor's mind jumped to taking a food history of myself. First year of life: baby formula, several rounds of antibiotics, and food mash. Childhood: home-cooked, traditional Chinese foods, but also more antibiotics, almost yearly, for bronchitis. Adolescence: a transition to the Standard American Diet, with regular meals from McDonald's and Jack in the Box, along with TV dinners and Lean Cuisines at home, and Hershey's chocolate bars and Pepperidge Farm frozen cakes as daily treats. I was currently eating a lot of prepackaged foods, too, for their convenience.

When I thought about the cocktail of pesticides, herbicides, plastics from food containers, tobacco residues, and other chemicals I had unknowingly ingested along with my food, my body tensed up. The catch-22 was that this kind of awareness could generate stress. So before I got too much further, an inner voice reminded me of my How to Get Off the Couch assignment and said, *Give yourself permission to receive. Receive this present positivity instead of dwelling on all that's wrong.* I opened my eyes to the girls clambering about the barn, and gave a little smile. The group around me was sipping their mugs of broth and swapping stories on urban farming, and I decided to join them. Before leaving, I went over to the retail pantry and bought some sauerkraut, a bottle of apple cider vinegar, and a bag of sea salt. I peeled the girls away from their play, drove home, and lay on the couch for an hour. Then I contemplated when to take my first stab at bone broth with the slow cooker.

David called the next day from wherever he was—I couldn't keep up with his schedule anymore—and I shared with him all I had learned, both as basic information every doctor should know, and also what to do for Rosa's teeth.

There was a brief silence at the other end.

"Hello?" I said.

"Changing the way you cook," he said, "and qigong and meditations and circadian gobbledygook—I can't keep up!"

David couldn't keep up with *me*?

The next day, as I was sitting in meditation, the golden fields appeared again. An endless swath of tall grasses swaying in the breeze. *Let intuition tell your thinking mind where to look next*, I reminded myself. I was trying, but my thinking mind was blank. The image was so clear, however, that I sent Pia an email asking her if she could make anything of it.

A few days later, she called.

"It's wheat," she said. "You're seeing golden fields of wheat."

"Really?"

"I can taste it!" Pia said, laughing.

"Why is wheat coming up? Could it be something else?"

"You know, I had a lot of trouble with my health until I went gluten-free. Maybe it has something to do with gluten?"

"Gluten? I thought the whole gluten-free thing was a fad."

I thanked her and immediately got online. My research told me that gluten is a protein in wheat, barley, and rye. In people who are genetically susceptible, gluten can trigger an autoimmune reaction in the gut called celiac disease. Although celiac disease is typically thought of as a "gut problem," more precisely, it is a body-wide inflammatory disease that manifests in the gut. Celiacs, it turns out, can have poor teeth for a couple of reasons. One, gut inflammation can lead to poor absorption of minerals, making the teeth generally weaker and prone to decay. And two, enamel defects commonly seen in celiacs make teeth vulnerable to cavity-forming bacteria.

In children, celiac disease often presents as failure to thrive, anemia, digestive symptoms like diarrhea or constipation, or a distinctive rash on the skin. Rosa was too healthy. She had hit every milestone in her development, and her height and weight were above average for her age group. She had no signs or symptoms of anemia, digestive symptoms, or rashes. But in addition to her cavities, she did have another symptom common to celiacs: frequent canker sores.

Then I started wondering about myself. While the incidence of celiac disease in the Chinese was only a small percentage of the 1 percent of Americans who have the disease, the searches for gluten kept citing a familiar name: Hashimoto's thyroiditis. For those who had the genes, gluten could trigger Hashimoto's thyroiditis, which was basically the same as postpartum thyroiditis. The connection was so well-established that celiac experts routinely screened their patients for Hashimoto's. So why wasn't the reverse happening? My endocrinologist, a leading expert, hadn't mentioned it at all, and I had asked him point blank if there was anything I could do to lessen the risk of another flare-up. I understood how doctors were trained—he had been focused on treating the end-effects of the disease with drugs. But what about addressing potential root causes as a form of treatment?

In addition to celiac disease, there was mounting literature on "non-celiac gluten sensitivity," or NCGS, which includes a wide spectrum of conditions from simple digestive intolerance to autoimmune attacks in the nervous system that cause vertigo, mood swings, migraines, and seizures. Another article spoke of gluten triggering inflammation in the brain, which in turn increased anxiety and hypersensitivity. If gluten was causing my dizziness or hypersensitivity or fatigue, might removing it help?

The ancestral diet contained grains, including gluten—it preferred ancient varieties of wheat and rye to modern hybrids, and it preferred soaked or fermented preparations over ones that refined and bleached. So I had to learn which foods were gluten-free. Searching for "gluten-free diet," I scrolled…and scrolled…and scrolled some more. The list of gluten-containing foods looked as infinite as the golden fields of wheat stretching out to the horizon.

I shut my laptop down, pretended like I hadn't seen it, and moved on to easier things.

Like bone broth.

I called David down to assist me in the kitchen. The two pounds of raw chicken feet and necks got him interested. We rinsed them, dumped them into the slow cooker, then added two tablespoons of raw apple cider vinegar. A dash of sea salt, and filtered water to the rim, and we were done. Just wait two days.

Returning the apple cider vinegar to the cabinet, I noted an extra-large bottle of soy sauce. It was on the gluten list, so I pulled it out. I opened the fridge and noted the barbecue sauce, hoisin sauce, and beer. In the pantry, there was pasta, crackers, couscous, different kinds of flours, and cereals. Gluten was lurking everywhere! How could I live my life with more relaxation if I had to navigate the gluten maze?

Before jumping to conclusions, I needed proof. David and Sonia didn't have any symptoms that warranted testing, so Rosa and I would get tested. In the meantime, I grabbed a slice of country batard from the bread basket and enjoyed it as I never had before.

Please, let the tests be negative, I thought.

Two weeks later, the results arrived in the mail. For both Rosa and me, the celiac genes were negative. I exhaled deeply. Then I read on. Another set of genes was positive. The interpretative note read: *possible increased risk for NCGS,* or a general gluten sensitivity. And as for the antibodies, both Rosa and I had tested positive for two things: (1) antibodies against gluten, and (2) antibodies against our own tissues. This meant that eating gluten caused our immune system to atta cells within our own bodies—in other words, gluten triggered autoimmunity.

By now, I was used to the paradoxical responses of both relief and disbelief. But I felt a grief that was new. It was for Rosa. For me to eliminate a whole class of foods felt cumbersome but necessary. For my daughter to do so, at the age of five, felt unjust.

The next day, Rosa got the first set of cavities filled.

The week after, the next set.

Afterward, Rosa was at home, playing with a ball of Play-Doh she had picked from the dentist's toy chest. I sat down next to her, told her how brave she had been with the cavities, and decided to share with her the news on gluten.

"There are some foods you can't eat anymore. We'll try to do this as a family. For now, it's important that you only eat food that Daddy or I give you, okay? It's like an allergy."

"Allergy?" she said, glancing at me, then grabbing her Play-Doh. She rolled it, pounded it flat, and poked her finger through it.

"It's something called gluten...it's in a lot of breads and crackers and pasta...sorta like Sonia's allergies to cats, except you don't get itchy and sneezy. You get cavities and little sores in your mouth, and maybe some other boo-boos we can't see."

"Gloot-in,'" she repeated.

"I'm allergic, too," I said. "We'll be allergic together. Just like Daddy and Sonia are allergic to cats together."

Rosa giggled, repeating *gloot-in*, and scampered off. I put the Play-Doh away, realizing, *Wait, it contains gluten!* I had most of the list memorized by now. I tossed it in the trash, hoping I wasn't tossing out Rosa's chance at a normal childhood, too.

For the next month, we embarked on a family experiment. We would eliminate gluten, yes, but we would go beyond just that. Having researched gut-healing diets, we decided to remove gluten, dairy, and all grains for thirty days, filling in the gaps with nutrient-dense, ancestrally prepared foods. To cope, we tried to see the humor in all this. I reminded David that chocolate ice cream was out on two counts—it contained dairy and was nutrient-poor. He reminded me the same was true for

Milk Duds. Another one of his jokes was "Gluten-free, dairy-free, and taste-free."

"*Not* taste-free," I would counter. I was still the primary cook in the family, and this diet was a challenge to try new recipes, focusing primarily on taste. Over time, I would realize they weren't mutually exclusive. Nutrient-dense equaled flavor-dense.

Day one of our family experiment: A hard day of cooking and sorting foods, but otherwise peaceful.

Day two. The same.

Day three. Everyone was fine, except for me. My gut had revolted. The once-a-day formed stool turned into five-times-a-day diarrhea. Horrible cramps. Painful gas. Sleep once again interrupted throughout the night. I remembered that I'd had an intense withdrawal after my initial acupuncture treatment, and that the payoff was worth it, so I reminded myself to hang tight, and 8: *Inhabit your body.* But my mind wanted to detach, and to give up on this crazy diet. Desperate, I tried Master Gu's sound healing practice, with a focus on stirring up my digestive system. *Ganggg...ganggg...ganggg...! Fooo...fooo...fooo...!* Multiple times a day, every day.

My body's rebellion continued for five or six days, and then my digestion calmed down. Over the coming months, we stayed gluten-free and nutrient-dense, but added back some grains. And our whole family experienced a shift in health that no randomized, placebo-controlled trial could ever capture. The responses were simply too individual, and the symptoms too disparate.

First, I rose to 5.5–6.0 on the functionality scale. On average, I could do five hours a day of light work, getting outside on most days, though still needing rest periods. My sleep was still up and down, but when I was able to sleep, it felt deeper and more refreshing. The dizziness lessened a notch, presumably because there was less inflammation in my brain and gut. The hypersensitivity to sounds and light lessened, and I began listening to the radio more often. As a result, I didn't have to do my qigong practices as rigidly, or do acupuncture every month, and my circadian routine was now more forgiving. I often forgot when I was supposed to do what, and by not having to stick so closely to an hour-by-hour schedule, an inner sense of freedom grew.

Most remarkable was my thyroid. The full replacement dose of thyroid supplement I had been taking for two years soon became too strong, and I would taper down from 100 to 25 micrograms, the lowest maintenance dose. The inflammation in my thyroid must have diminished and therefore allowed for healing, and in its healing, it began to make its own thyroid hormones again. So what I had learned in medical school, that autoimmunity isn't reversible, wasn't, in fact, true.

As for Rosa, her cavities stopped forming. Other symptoms, things we had written off as mere idiosyncrasies, also resolved. Like her karate kicks at night: Rosa went from being an active sleeper to a sound sleeper. And her proclivity for drama: her moods became more stable. The pains on her shins, which we had been erroneously calling "growing pains," resolved, and the canker sores in her mouth became less frequent.

As for Sonia, her two minor but persistent afflictions—wheezing with colds, and the persistent rash around her lips—both resolved within a few months.

Even David noted some changes. A few pounds came off, most visibly around his waist, and his post-lunch energy crashes disappeared. Mostly, he just felt better. It was subtle, but when we were closing in on six months on the gluten-free, ancestral diet, David said one morning, "Wow, I've got a lot more energy these days!"

"*More* energy?" I smiled, gritting my teeth.

9. Heal the gut.

TWENTY ONE

2011

After the dietary changes, my body felt stronger, but also a little alien. Like the low-grade buzz of electricity in buildings that suddenly goes quiet during a power outage, my body felt quiet without the background inflammation. It probably should have felt peaceful, but instead, I felt uneasy; the buzz had been there for so long, and without it, my inner workings didn't quite know how to function. There seemed to be a void.

David was appointed to California's primary energy agency, based in Sacramento, eighty miles northeast of Berkeley. He stayed there Mondays through Thursdays, and was home Fridays and the weekends. Thankfully, I had the support of David's parents and Dolma, plus an increasing number of neighbors and friends we knew and trusted. Once I got a sense of where my energy was and got the logistics sorted out, this arrangement, though a big adjustment, proved favorable for David and me. We had some natural space built into our marriage now, and it took the pressure off our differences in tempo and energy. Unexpectedly, David found he wanted more downtime when he was home; whereas I found, with my increased cooking skills and more room in our new home, I enjoyed having friends and family over. I also found that I missed him—both his emotional and physical presence—which awakened a part of me I had thought was dead.

This realization came to me one morning, as I was doing my visualizations. The girls had helped me convert an unused walk-in closet into my meditation room—"The Quiet Room," the girls, years later, would name it, making it over with decorations and paints. I threw a floor pillow on top of a small rug, and on a mini-bookshelf I put an assortment of things dear to me: a couple of pine cones from a trip to the Adirondacks with David, a few abalone shell fragments from our wedding day, dried lavender for its scent, some arts and crafts from

Rosa and Sonia, and a pewter stand with a single white taper candle, given to me by my godfather.

That morning, I lit the candle, gazed into the single flame, and after a few minutes, I began to see something in my mind's eye. It was me, sitting as I was, cross-legged on the pillow. In my center was a round shadow—the void I had been feeling. And within that black void was another round shadow, hardly bigger than a speck. It was orange. A tiny, translucent sun. The tiny sun seemed to pulsate, as though trying to fill the blackness. But it was stuck, unable to expand.

I felt this orange circle might represent pleasure or passion. Somewhere along the corkscrew path, the shadows of grief and pain had obliterated my capacity for pleasure. Sure, I could still laugh with the girls or joke around with David or feel the sacredness in my sanctuaries, but the pleasure I was missing was something rawer, more lasting. Hands over my navel, I wondered, *What do I long for?* More erotic passion? More restorative in-between spaces? More permanence in a world of constant change? Perhaps I was longing for *me*, to reconnect with my body in an organic way. Freely.

David wanted that for me, too. More than anything. His being away in Sacramento seemed to allow him to see me and my challenges more clearly, separate from how they challenged him. On the weekends, if I asked, "Can we just lie with each other tonight and enjoy snuggling without sex?" he would say "Sure," and not need to move to the other room. I felt bolder in setting my boundaries without guilt; he felt bolder in voicing his vulnerabilities. One night in bed, he said, "I know you think I'm always pushing for us to have more sex, and you think I don't appreciate the sex we do have." His voice was husky, practically a whisper. "You know, it's hard on my end, too, feeling like my partner doesn't want me."

I saw for the first time his loneliness in not having felt wanted, and it pained me. "It's not you, really. I love you. I just don't feel any desire at all." I stroked his arm. "But I really want to want you again."

He looked up. "You do?"

"I do."

I didn't know how to approach the act of reclaiming desire. My new learner's mind was a blank, so I read through my How to Get Off the Couch list for pointers. 8. *Inhabit your body* was obvious. But how? Qigong, maybe? It felt awkward and contrived to approach desire with a disciplined practice like that. But if qigong helped to activate freer-flowing energy in general, and passion was a type of energy, why couldn't it activate freer-flowing passion?

The science of pleasure showed that certain practices can increase levels of dopamine, the key chemical involved in motivation and pleasure. Dopamine is what creates the highs we experience during intense workouts, or during sex. Deficiencies in this chemical, then, can lead to fatigue, sleep troubles, poor mood, and foggy thinking. Interested in natural ways to boost dopamine, I returned to a concept I had learned in medical school. The dopamine pathway works by priming, or conditioning responses, so that the release of dopamine triggers the release of yet more dopamine, which is why repetitive small acts of pleasure are also dopamine-producing. Given enough repetition, the neural pathways of arousal become heartier—the principle of neuroplasticity—and given enough repetition, the genes for pleasure might also turn back on—the principle of epigenetics.

This was enough for me to commit to doing the "deer exercise," a qigong practice that touted benefits to core sexuality and overall vitality. Sit naked in front of a mirror, the website said. So I made sure I had total privacy, locked the door, then got undressed. I grabbed a pillow and sat in front of the full-length mirror in our closet. Take a good look at yourself, the website said, Notice your body, and feel your sexuality. I tried and felt nothing, not even a hint of the tiny sun within. But I also remembered how nothing had come up the many times I first attempted the visualizations Pia had taught me. Like the visualizations, and like the standard qigong practice, this was a *practice.* So I continued on.

Choose a mantra, the website said, any phrase that expresses self-love or self-possession. "I am beautiful," I said, looking at my naked self. Traces of the Gorgon were there. My hair was coarse and sprouting its first grays. My forehead bore fine lines, and the crow's feet next to my eyelids were deeper. Dark circles underlined my eyes. Before I got too deflated, I moved on to the next steps, which were to contract the vaginal muscles while relaxing the abdomen.

I contracted, then relaxed.

Contracted, then relaxed.

I did a round of twenty contractions and relaxations.

Waited.

Another around of twenty.

With each contraction, I imagined the mitochondrial powerhouses in my groin revving up their generators and sounding the horns to get the rusty engines working again. If I could get my reproductive organs humming, I wondered if I would be able to feel an organic sense of pleasure. At some point, Rosa and Sonia started banging on the bedroom door, asking to come in. I took one last look at my body, said "I am beautiful," and scanned it for my lost womanhood.

I practiced the deer exercise for months, sometimes in lieu of the traditional qigong practice, sometimes in addition to it. I came to see some signs of a truer me, beneath the Gorgon. My cheekbones were high like my mother's, and like her mother's. My long torso and legs were my father's, as was the wave in my hair and the dimple in my right cheek. My eyes and brows were a mix of the two. My posture, from the hundred-plus qigong practices telling me to hold my shoulders tall and not slouch into a smaller self, produced an almost regal silhouette. I could see how some might have thought me attractive once. During a practice on a day when I was feeling generally softer toward myself, I would stroke my arms, as I might have done with Rosa or Sonia. The feet I had judged too big, the buttocks and chest that were too flat, the hips that were too wide after pregnancy—perhaps the dopamine really was kicking in, because I was so tired of listening to these negative thoughts.

As I cast them out, a warmth radiated from my center. From that warmth came a deep appreciation of what my body had done for me. It had received considerable neglect in the form of processed and fast foods, rounds and rounds of antibiotics, and all the times I pushed past my aches and pains rather than listening to what my body was trying to say through them. My body had also sustained me through the boot camp of medical training, as well as two pregnancies, the second a very difficult one, and it was still persevering now. For so long I had treated it as a vessel to be used, or as a vessel that had let me down. In actuality, it was a vessel to be tended, to be honored, to be beheld.

The deer exercise began to feel good, as though blood and sensation were returning to my pelvis, and in this new flow, the tiny sun seemed to be growing, filling the void in my center. Like the functionality scale, it wasn't a stable fullness, but a waxing and waning one, whose overall long-term trajectory was toward expansion. The more I practiced, the more stable it became.

Whether it was the dopamine or a renewed self-possession, I came to feel younger than my now-forty-one-year-old self, by roughly five or six years. Taking 7: *Change your thoughts, change your genes* a few steps further, David and I decided to change our surroundings to match the earlier times when I was naturally aroused in play or sex, thinking it might help activate the pleasure pathways and genes. We switched sides of the bed, back to our old go-to sides. I took down the black-and-white poster of a city skyline next to my (new) side of the bed, and hung up a color photo of white butterflies fluttering about a royal blue sky, a photo from my college days. Since I was tolerating the TV and stereo more, we watched throwbacks from the '80s and '90s, like *The Breakfast Club, The Princess Bride, Splash.* As I cooked, I often played, in the background, Duran Duran or Erasure, my favorite hits from college and medical school. Soon, in lieu of the deer practice, I was dancing naked in front of the mirror to When In Rome's "The Promise," feeling twenty all over again.

David joined me in other ways. Living as a bachelor in Sacramento during the week gave him an appreciation for all that went into keeping the house and children, and to his credit, he chipped in more on the weekends. He put up a sticker on our bedroom mirror that said COOK— CLEAN—SLOW DOWN, to remind him of what I needed to feel loved. One Saturday, he asked where the vacuum cleaner was.

I smiled, amused instead of angry upon realizing he hadn't used it once. "Um, it's been in the same closet for over a year."

"Tell me where it is."

"I'll give you a hint—it's in a major closet that we open almost every day."

He found it and vacuumed the living room.

Over time, however, the differences between us became clearer. He could walk into a room where several dirty socks were strewn about, and truly not notice them. He could give the girls a bath, or take one himself, and truly not notice the ring of soap scum clinging to the tub. He would wash the dishes with the goal of getting them done, as opposed to getting them clean. So while I told him I was grateful, inwardly I excused him, letting go of my expectations.

I also started to reevaluate my own behavior. David had often said that I wanted things perfect around the house. Was that true? One morning, as I was about to make the bed, I thought, *Why is it so darn important that I make this bed?* Letting go of any perfectionism, I asked myself, *Do I really care?* And surprisingly, I didn't. My father had instilled this habit into my siblings and me as something he learned from his military days, a habit that started the day off in good working order. And for years, decades, that was how it had worked for me. But did I need to do it now? No. I had also made my bed when I was young because it saved me from being disciplined. Was this an issue now? No. I did prefer the house tidy, because I didn't like clutter, and I didn't like to spend time looking for lost items. But was this an issue with the bed? No. In a burst of playfulness, I rustled up the bed linens and marched out of the bedroom.

It was beyond playful. I felt emancipated! I stopped making the bed altogether, and took pleasure in seeing it messy. This lasted a whole of three weeks, because on a certain Saturday, I was retiring to our room, ready to climb into our messy bed and fluff up my lumpy pillow when I saw the comforter tucked in and the pillows fluffed.

"Who—?" I said.

"Who what?" David said, confused.

"Who made the bed?"

"It wasn't made, so I made it after breakfast."

I flopped onto the bed and laugh-cried.

After David brushed his teeth, I asked him to get naked, and then *he* started to laugh-cry.

"Who—?" he said.

I shushed him and grabbed a couple of small pouches from the nightstand drawer. They were secret purchases from Good Vibrations, an adult toy store I had visited a few days earlier.

"Wanna?" I whispered, thinking he would be ecstatic. But he lay next to me, unsure what to do. "To kick-start my pleasure centers, we've gotta spice up our sex life."

"What about your dizziness and stuff?"

"I'll be careful with my body."

He still lay there, not making any moves.

"Don't be so shy," I joked, nudging him. It was the first time I had ever seen him self-conscious. "Don't be so sensitive," I joked again, reveling in the role reversal.

We made love with the aid of some creative toys.

When all was said and done, David said, "Who do I have to thank for this?"

"You have *you* to thank."

His making the bed had somehow made me feel seen. To feel seen was to feel wanted, though until then, I hadn't been able to pinpoint that I wasn't feeling wanted either. To know that David didn't just want sex, that he wanted *me*—which I understood now because I was in a more self-possessed place, and believed I was wantable—it was better than any dopamine-boosting drug could ever achieve.

I lay staring at the ceiling, feeling a deep satisfaction. Not about achieving raw pleasure, because that didn't happen right away. But about sex no longer feeling like an item on my mental to-do list. I was engaging simply because I wanted to.

A dreamless sleep came over me.

10. Break old habits that no longer serve you.

11. Practice pleasure. It's serious work.

TWENTY TWO

2012

Another year of integration and consolidation passed.

I only saw Bob for acupuncture now on an as-needed basis, every two or three months. Though I stayed at the level of 5.5–6.0 on the scale, I gained more flexibility with regard to my circadian routines. I continued taking my supplements, watching my diet, and taking my walks. The most measurable change during this time was my intuition. Many of my dreams were infused with celestial motifs: golden whales doing flips high in the air; elevator rides to the penthouse of a hotel; a spaceship that flew to the heavens; intimate exchanges with larger-than-human people with perfect faces and rounded features, which, upon waking, I thought might have represented angels. Odd electrical phenomena began to happen, where lights would surge in intensity during my meditations, or outgoing calls would be made from our landline without anyone having made them. Once, in the middle of the night, two police officers knocked on our door because they received a call from our house.

I was both fascinated and freaked out by what was happening, but David felt there had to be a rationale. To me, it felt like more than just a heightened awareness of things that had been happening all along. When we couldn't find a mechanical explanation, I attributed the occurrences to quantum physics, or lightheartedly to Yoda and the Force, refraining from labeling them as "good" or "bad." Just "interesting."

But why now, and increasingly so? It all seemed to correlate with my qigong and intuition practices. I wasn't sure what to do. I didn't want to stop, since these practices were helping me to heal. As I thought about it, I wanted someone to guide me in intuition, but more specifically with regard to health, both mine and others'. In characteristic form, David mentioned this to a friend in the sustainability field. She recommended I contact Martine Bloquiaux, a friend of hers who might assuage some of my anxieties and teach me medical intuition.

Martine had grown up in Belgium in a family of doctors and nurses. At a young age, she could see what she later understood as diseases in people's bodies. Later in life, after having studied international law and with the support of her father, a general surgeon, she decided to use her intuitive gifts for healing. She took various integrative medicine courses and studied with healers in Asia and Europe, learning how to translate into physiological and anatomical terms what she was seeing.

I reached out to Martine with my mixed bag of emotions. First off, she reassured me that these phenomena are common to anyone who becomes more attuned. Second, she told me to ground myself in ordinary life with David and the girls, and in my body. Third, she taught me something new to harness my newfound energies: ask yes-no questions when holding a health concern in meditation.

I began to play around with this. The key was to tune in to my body and detect any sensations I felt. Soon, I "calibrated" a pressure in my forehead to mean yes, and an absence of one to mean no. Initially, I asked questions about my own health, simple questions like "Is this an ideal dose of vitamin C?" or "Am I sensitive to dairy?" Then, when a friend emailed asking about his gout, I held the question of which joint was affected ("Is it his ankle, yes or no?") and on which side of the body ("Is it on the right side, yes or no?"). When my mother called saying her primary doctor found elevated inflammatory markers that put her at risk for heart attacks and strokes, I tried to decipher why ("Does she have an infection somewhere, yes or no?" "Does she have inflammation in her mouth, yes or no?"). I began to do this almost every day, following up my intuitive answers with a good H&P, reviewing whatever labs or other concrete evidence my friends and family had, and always sticking to low-risk cases. I found that, if I could keep my rational mind from butting in too early, I was getting faster and more accurate. It was wild! Since my doctor's mind couldn't well explain it, I rationalized it by saying I was abiding by a modified scientific method: *Ask a question* → *Skip a couple steps* → *Conduct an experiment.*

The big question I held in meditation was whether I was ready to start working with patients again. I got a strong yes. So I consulted with my logical mind, too. To accommodate my energy, I knew I had to start with a reduced schedule, like ten or fifteen hours a week, then build it out as I was able. I also knew I couldn't return to how I used to practice medicine. I had learned too much along my own journey about its limitations and potential failings.

I had to find a brave new way.

For a few months, I explored the different fields within integrative medicine—an umbrella term for anything from old-fashioned family practice doctors who prescribe ancestral diets and lifestyle; to doctors who supplement primary care with medical acupuncture; to multidisciplinary clinics with classes for yoga, mindfulness-based stress reduction, and nutrition; to doctors who prescribe anti-aging hormone therapies or electromagnetic machines to improve circulation; and everything in between. I contacted and shadowed a handful of local doctors, trying to find my niche. My last stop was Dr. Julia Getzelman, an integrative pediatrician in a small group practice in San Francisco. When I told her what I was interested in, she asked, "Have you looked into functional medicine?"

I hadn't heard of it.

Functional, Dr. Getzelman explained, referred to the capacity of the mind and body to perform optimally. In functional medicine, dysfunctions are understood to be the result of lifelong imbalances between a person's environment and his or her genes. Left uncorrected, these dysfunctions can reach a threshold beyond which symptoms or diseases manifest. Functional medicine helps clinicians identify and address a person's dysfunctions, to restore health. While the science in functional medicine is cutting-edge, its philosophies are a synthesis of ancient practices, like those of traditional Chinese medicine or Ayurveda. The approach is based on systems, looking at the body as a whole within a larger whole. It sounded like a readymade framework of what I had been working piecemeal toward in my n of 1 journey—but applicable to an n of many.

I couldn't wait.

In the fall, I was sitting on the edge of my bed in a hotel room in Santa Monica, California. I had made it to the five-day foundational course sponsored by the Institute for Functional Medicine. Uncertain of how I would fare with travel, I had arrived a day early, and I was glad for it. The flight, though only an hour, had kicked up my dizziness. I'd spent the previous day drinking salty water, resting, stocking up on foods I could eat, resting some more, and getting in an extra practice of qigong. It was hardly the ease with which I once traveled the world, taking planes as though they were buses, hop-on, hop-off, and eating whatever the locals ate. I was determined, though, not to fall prey to anxiety or self-pity.

This morning I woke in better shape, grateful I could be here at all. I finished an early-morning meditation, got dressed and went down to the auditorium. There was a breakfast buffet table in the lobby. I didn't imagine I would find much I could eat, but the foods were meticulously labeled. There were coconut milk yogurts, grainless granola made of sprouted seeds and nuts, a wide assortment of fruit, hard-boiled eggs, organic coffees, and herbal teas (in other words, gluten- and dairy-free, but not taste-free). I piled my small plate full of nutrient-dense goodness and topped it off with a strawberry. Before eight in the morning, I was already liking functional medicine a whole lot.

The air in the auditorium was electric. Pop music played in the background as some three hundred health care professionals fiercely networked. From the badges I scanned, I estimated roughly half to be doctors, the other half made up of nutritionists, chiropractors, psychologists, acupuncturists, and other health care professionals, from all over the world. I picked a seat toward the right side, and introduced myself to the participants next to me, both doctors from my hometown of Austin, Texas, who had attended numerous functional medicine conferences. We caught up on the Austin music scene and the famous bats living under a bridge there. Then I closed my eyes, focused on my breath, and tried to keep my inner workings calm amidst all the stimulation.

When the lights dimmed and the music faded, a tall, slender man in a dark suit sprang onto the stage. This was Dr. Mark Hyman, a spokesperson and bestselling author in the field. He held a clicker in one hand and a bottle of water in the other, and wore a headset. Three large screens projected the first slide, its graphics stylish but not over the top. With Dr. Hyman starting to pace the stage, I felt like I was sitting in a TED talk rather than a medical conference. He welcomed us, then said, "This week you'll hear a lot of new information. You'll also hear old information presented in new ways. So I invite you to suspend disbelief and keep an open mind."

Well-versed in suspending disbelief now, I found myself nodding along.

"Most of you are here because you think the way we've learned medicine doesn't answer all the questions we have, or because your patients aren't getting better." With an easy smile, Dr. Hyman continued to pace the stage. "We're trained to be super-specialists, but in today's world of complex diseases, we need to be super-generalists. And to be super-generalists, we need to understand inflammation inside and out."

I typed my notes on my laptop, reverting back to my medical school days of list upon cherished list to condense the masses of information. The two most important lists were:

The Five Causes of Disease

1. Infections

2. Allergens

3. Toxins

4. Stress (emotional, mental, or physical)

5. Poor diet

The Seven Essential Ingredients of Optimal Health

1. Real food

2. Hormonal balance

3. A healthy environment (water, air, light)

4. Relaxation and pleasure

5. Adequate sleep

6. Exercise or movement

7. Community, love, purpose

This paradigm had amazing overlap with the Ecological Paradigm of Health, but was adapted to individuals and organized in an easy-to-apply format. What mattered were the presence of any or all causes, the absence of essential ingredients, and the capacity of these factors to interact synergistically. The individual mattered, too, because the same factors could affect different people differently. Two individuals could share a diagnosis (obesity, for example), but the causes and deficiencies in one person (say, allergens and a lack of exercise) might differ from those in the next person (say, pollutants, emotional trauma, and inadequate sleep). Alternatively, the same deficiency (magnesium, for example) could cause different symptoms or diseases in different people (high blood pressure in one person, migraines in another). The greater the number of causes or deficiencies, the greater the damage to the cells, the more serious the disease, and the harder the task of achieving optimal health.

In simplified terms, small things can multiply to cause big disease.

The doctor's role, Dr. Hyman continued, was to identify and treat whichever of these factors was an issue for any given patient—and it all started with gut health. Without a well-functioning digestive system, we can't digest nutrients from food, much less absorb or use them. He covered a lot of the material I had learned earlier about the gut flora and its importance in metabolism, hormones, and overall health. But he added a 5R protocol for the healing of the gut (in addition to simply changing the diet): Remove—remove stresses, like processed foods or intestinal infections; Replace—replace herbs or enzymes to break food down better; Reinoculate—reinoculate with beneficial gut flora (like in fermented foods); Repair—repair the gut lining with key amino acids (like in bone broth!) and antioxidants (like vitamin C—in oranges!);

Rebalance—rebalance sleep, stress, and exercise (like the circadian routine). By addressing the 5Rs, healing the gut might not take nearly as long as it had for me.

Next, he talked about supplements. How the quality matters. How there are companies that undergo independent testing to ensure a higher standard. How high-potency vitamins, minerals, herbs, and amino acids can accelerate the healing process. How most people can stand to replete their vitamin D, magnesium, and B-complex, but this is especially important in addressing chronic health challenges. How these nutrients are key players in restoring the immune system's function, dampening inflammation, healing the brain, and supporting detoxification in the body. And how a good diet is always the best way to go, but many people need higher doses of certain nutrients than they can get from foods, and some people can't manage an elimination diet right off the bat.

Just before the break, he talked about detoxification. This is the body's natural process of removing toxins, or any substance that can cause cell injury and disease. Toxins include internal waste from our own metabolic processes, as well as external waste from drugs, pollutants, harmful germs, or radiation. The primary detox organ is the liver, but there are accessory detox organs, too: a healthy gut rids our bodies of waste via stool; the skin via sweat; the lungs via mucus and exhalation; the kidneys via urine; and the immune system via lymphatic channels.

The only way I had known before to reduce pollutants in the body was to live a clean life and eat a nutrient-dense diet. Though still important to reduce harmful chemicals, for myself and for the planet, certain foods and nutrients could help my body more efficiently metabolize and eliminate harmful substances. That is, in addition to 5: *Detoxify the house*, we can detoxify our bodies—*(and detoxify yourself)*.

Break time. People stood up and stretched. My fingers were stiff from typing, and a flu-like malaise was simmering in my chest, likely triggered by the fast-paced talk, the bright stage lights, and the new environment. So I stood up and stretched, too, then took the elevator to my hotel room. I plopped onto the freshly made linens, and chilled out until I was motivated enough for some sound healing qigong. *Xin…xin…xin…* I had done this practice so many times that the effects were almost immediate, and my symptoms slipped away as if beads of sweat off my forehead.

More at ease, I called home.

Rosa answered. "Where are you, Mommy?"

Sonia hollered in the background, "Mama!" They were used to David taking business trips or holidays, but not me. I asked Rosa to put me on speaker phone.

"I'm learning how to be a better doctor," I said.

"But you da whole best doctah in da whole wide world," Sonia said, now four and full of words.

I laughed. "There's a whole lot I don't know, and there's even more that I'll never know."

David chimed in. "Hey, hon. How's the conference?"

"Incredible. I'm learning so much my head is literally starting to spin."

"I love hearing that," David said, straining over the background noise. The girls sounded as though they had scampered off into the next room, where they were now hollering and making a general ruckus. "Girls!" he shouted, taking the phone off speaker. Something sounded as though it smashed into a hundred pieces. "Oh, gotta go!" Click.

I plopped onto the bed, smiling. I wanted to know, I didn't want to know.

A few minutes after eleven, after an extra-long break, I returned to the auditorium. The next session was well underway, and the speaker was talking about oft-overlooked root causes of common conditions. "We often treat the symptoms," he said, "without looking further into what's causing the condition. That's like treating an overflowing sink by mopping up the floor instead of removing the clog." The "clogs" were none other than the Five Causes of Disease from Dr. Hyman's presentation. By addressing any or all of these clogs, we could restore flow to the sink. Just as in traditional Chinese medicine, in the functional approach, disease is healed by removing the obstructions.

The speaker then honed in on infections as a cause, explaining that many are "stealth infections," those low-grade enough that they don't manifest like the typical acute infection—a cold or pneumonia or gastroenteritis. Bacteria and viruses can reside within the human body and cause just enough trouble to activate the immune system and rouse inflammation, but not enough to cause an overt infection or necessarily show up on routine screening tests.

This was a radical notion that challenged the dominant ideas around infections. I was still trying to decide what to make of it when he flipped through multiple slides showing current and past research to support this notion: archaic bacteria that could cause symptoms of irritable bowel syndrome if they overgrew in the small intestine; molds found in patients with Alzheimer's; viruses that cause chronic fatigue as well as autoimmune thyroiditis.

During the lunch break, I grabbed my lunch to go and returned to my room. I wanted to rest, but more, I wanted to review the slides on stealth infections and chronic fatigue. Epstein-Barr virus, or EBV, could cause chronic fatigue, as well as dysautonomia. Lyme and other tick-borne infections could, too. Though I wasn't aware of having had any tick bites in my life, I knew I had contracted EBV during my second year of residency. They were a miserable few months.

It was thirteen years earlier, shortly after Kurt had died. I woke before dawn for my ER shift. My body felt as hot as an oven, my throat was raw, and the glands in my neck were tender. I called in sick and slept the entire day, as well as the next, and the next. The fever subsided, but for the next month, I was slogging through my ER rotation. "God, Cynthia," one of my co-residents said, "you've been lookin' so haggard, you should get screened for mono." I tested positive. The diagnosis didn't change anything, because as I understood it then, waiting it out and resting was all I could do. Three months down the line, I recovered. I had assumed this meant forever.

The reality was, after acute mono resolves, EBV hibernates in white blood cells. For a lot of people, hibernation lasts forever. But when the immune system becomes suppressed or dysfunctional (like from chronic stress, shift work, nutritional deficiencies, or gut inflammation), viruses like EBV can rise up and throw a "reactivation" party. Reactivation can be sustained, and can cause chronic fatigue, brain fog, achy muscles and joints, and dizziness. There were several centers around the world that studied EBV and chronic fatigue, including Stanford. I found some studies of doctors in those clinics treating such patients with antiviral medication for several months; many experienced reductions in their viral numbers and an improvement in their quality of life.

As I closed down my laptop, I reflected on EBV and other potential root causes in my case. What if, I wondered, I had known about functional medicine years earlier and removed any of the five root causes, restoring the seven essential ingredients to optimal health? Might I have compressed my healing time by months or years? Might I have averted the sudden disturbance in Beijing and its grueling aftermath altogether? Looking back and risking regret was something I tried to avoid. But suddenly I became nostalgic for a life that could have been.

12. Investigate hidden root causes.

Over the course of the conference, I learned much more. It wasn't all dense science. There were clinical practice tools, too. How to solicit the patient's health goals, which is qualitatively different than asking for their "chief complaints." How to take a patient history using a timeline chart, including the parents' and grandparents' histories (genetics and epigenetics), so that, at a glance, the patient and doctor can understand why his or her health challenges developed. How to organize, in chart form, the various systems' imbalances. How to prioritize which tests and which protocols to do when. How to enlist the patient in the treatment plan, so the doctor-patient relationship becomes a partnership. Then there were the how-tos of protocols: detox, core food plans, elimination diets. One session was a detailed physical exam, focused solely on the mouth. For an hour, we learned how to evaluate the teeth, palate, tongue, tonsils, and gums for nutritional deficiencies, inflammation, and infections. This added whole new dimensions to the basic H&P.

In his closing remarks, Dr. Hyman summarized the highlights of the week. It was clear to me that this was *deep* medicine, diving into the root causes of disease. *Slow* medicine, recognizing the primacy of the patient-doctor relationship and its role in healing. And *real* medicine, evaluating the body as a dynamic, interconnected web of systems.

He concluded by playing a video testimonial of one of his young patients, a girl who looked to be roughly seven—Rosa's age—who had been on steroids for horrible rashes and other autoimmune issues. She declared how well she felt after eliminating gluten and dairy and processed foods, clearing her body of toxins, and tapering off her steroids and other medications. She spoke of how Dr. Hyman and functional medicine would give her a chance at being a healthy teenager.

I can't recall any specific phrases she said, or any specific therapies she named. What stuck with me was her innocence, her right to health. She moved me out of my doctor's mind and into the healer's heart. *This* was why I was here, I thought. Sure, I could take away loads of new and emerging science. But the millions who were suffering, loudly and silently, and whose suffering I now understood from my own journey on the corkscrew path—they had been my original calling to be a doctor. There had been so many ailments I hadn't had the tools to address. But here was the possibility of integrating whole-foods diets and ancient wisdom with root-cause paradigms and the best of Western medicine. And I couldn't forget the intuition, which would help me navigate this new roadmap.

Deep in my chest, I felt a strong and steady *lub-dub, lub-dub*. My original calling was still beating.

As I walked through the front door, Rosa and Sonia leapt into my arms. They had dressed up for the occasion—princess gowns, one yellow, the other blue, matching plastic high heels. David had a vegetable soup simmering on the stove. It was good to be home.

The next few days, I wasted no time in taking clinical pearls from the conference and trying them out. Me, my own test case.

I performed a detailed oral exam with a pen light in the mirror: upper gums inflamed (*mouth flora imbalances? generalized inflammation?*), midline fissure on the tongue (*deficiency in B vitamins?*).

I ordered several key supplements: magnesium, zinc, selenium, vitamins D and B-complex, Coenzyme Q 10, among others.

I also started making green smoothies: kale, dandelion leaf, parsley, lemon juice, and apples.

One morning, as I was reviewing which screening tests to order for EBV reactivation syndrome, my forehead tightened. A familiar pressure sensation. It tightened more. This was the first time I had noticed an attunement happening outside my meditation or qigong practice. Could it be that my intuition knew without my consciously accessing it, and that my left and right brains were integrating?

Sure enough, my labs came back positive. I called a doctor whom I had met at the functional medicine conference, an expert in chronic infections, and he wrote me a prescription. So I added antiviral drugs to my regimen.

A few days later, *wham.* Another major withdrawal reaction. Similar to post-acupuncture and post-elimination diet. I was back on the couch, this time for a week. Then two. During this time, I had recurring dreams of diving into a green lake, trying to reach the bottom, then realizing it was actually a cesspool. I would try to propel myself to the surface, but the filth was like a net over me. I would awaken, gasping for air, and it reminded me of the airlessness I used to feel when I crawled into my metaphorical shoebox. Was I clearing out the muck in my body? Or was I doing more harm than good with my regimen, and backtracking?

One night at three in the morning, I shuffled to the bathroom, waking David up.

"You okay?" he whispered.

"I dunno." I went to the bathroom, relieved myself, then crawled back in bed. "I keep telling myself to hang in there, that this is all par for the course." I pulled the covers over my head and grumbled, "I'm so sick and tired of this shit."

"What?"

I assumed he was going to tell me to be more hopeful. "Nothing, never mind."

"Did you say you're sick of this shit?"

"Yeah." My head was still buried under the covers.

"It's refreshing to hear you say that!"

I peered out. "It is?"

"You've been such a diligent doctor, Cynthia, and such a patient patient. But the truth is, this is fuckin' hard, and you rarely vent!" He rolled toward me. "Go ahead, punch me."

"I'm not gonna punch you."

"No, really. Pretend I'm your illness. Hit me as hard as you can."

I shook my head.

"I insist."

Okay, then. I threw off my covers and socked it to him.

"Yeah, baby! Again!"

I socked it to him harder. "This is fucking hard!" It was so cathartic, I threw an extra punch.

"*Yeeoowww*," David pleaded, like a wounded cat. "There's a lot of grief behind those punches!"

I kissed him and told him to go back to sleep. I stared up at the ceiling, wondering, *Was* there still a lot of grief in me? David had probably meant it as a passing comment, but it made me revisit the cesspool in my dreams. I knew the health impacts of grief. Grief not just as deep loss, but as disappointment, as anger, as shame. Like other emotional stresses, it can increase inflammation in the body and the brain, aggravate physical pain, and cause digestive distress. Reports of infections that developed after intense grief have been linked to its impacts on hormone and immune function. I understood now that there was conscious grief (like my profound sadness after Kurt died), as well as grief held in the body (like the trauma Bob had released from my uterus). But how could I access the subconscious grief? And where was this grief in the formula of genes + lifetime exposures?

I suppose I was assessing the need for a different kind of detox. A detox of the soul.

TWENTY THREE

2013

The following spring, I felt ready for a soul detox. I had recovered from the physical detox, and had completed several months of antiviral drugs. I was up to a 6.5–7.0 and felt clearer inside. The signaling between my hormones and brain chemicals felt crisper, making me feel less a puppet on strings, and more human. Still, the total effect was less robust than I had hoped for, and a persistent low-grade disequilibrium remained. I was convinced that there were invisible, inaccessible stresses I had to somehow confront.

While David got the girls ready for a day at the zoo one Saturday, I was prepping for a daylong grief ritual. This wasn't exactly something I was looking forward to—wrestling in the muddy realms of the soul with a group of strangers. At least with qigong and acupuncture, there was a long tradition connected to my Chinese heritage. Something familiar, if novel. Venturing into grief carried the same promise and perils as venturing into intuition—what strangeness might emerge along with the healing? And how would my body respond?

The ritual was held in Point Reyes, near where I had celebrated my fortieth birthday. I was still unable to drive on the freeway, so the organizer arranged a ride for me with a man who was roughly my age. He and I walked into a homey, brown-shingled building, then into a room full of thirty mostly gray-haired folks, seated in a circle.

The sun was streaming through a stained-glass window, casting red and blue mosaics onto the floor. In the middle of the circle was an altar of remembrance—framed photos of beloveds, flowers in vases, and some votives. Since I didn't know specifically what I was there to grieve, I had brought my white tapered candle on the pewter stand, the one from my closet-turned-meditation room, a gift from my godfather. It represented all that was sacred in my life.

Francis Weller, a psychotherapist trained in grief work, was sitting at one end of the circle, playing an African hand drum. After everyone had settled, he played for another five minutes or so, then stopped drumming and introduced himself. A therapist who practiced soul-centered psychotherapy, he had studied traditional cultures from around the world, from Native Americans to the !Kung of the Kalahari Desert and the Dagara of West Africa, and incorporated their wisdom into grief work. He wore khaki pants and a charcoal merino sweater; a tidy salt-and-pepper beard covered his chin. He caught me studying him, responded with a warm smile, then began again to play the drum. A woman with long brown hair and a kind face sat opposite him in the circle.

"We're the holders of this space," he said, introducing her as the co-leader. "We will hold the space, so your souls feel safer to emerge."

My foot bobbed up and down, in excitement and nervousness.

"It takes courage to be here," Francis said. He gave a short talk, quoting Carl Jung and reciting poems from Rilke, Rumi, and others I loved. This felt less foreign to me now. I took out my pocket journal to jot down some of his pearls of wisdom.

Grief wasn't a problem to be solved, Francis said, it was an experience to be witnessed. If a grieving person didn't have a witness—if he grieved privately—he risked depression. If he didn't grieve enough, he risked suppression. Both of these were common in the West. Our primary "sins" were amnesia and anesthesia—we forgot, and we went numb. To grieve deeply, we had to elicit the soul. The *shy* soul. It usually needed to be coaxed out of hiding.

He concluded his introduction with a list of his own.

The Five Kinds of Grief

1. What we have loved and lost.

2. The places in us that have not known love (our shadows).

3. The sorrows of the world.

4. What we expected and did not receive.

5. Ancestral grief.

I tried to wrap my head around these insights. They rang true as soon as he said them, but they were so counter to how my evangelical upbringing, the medical culture, and the culture at large handled grief that I couldn't figure out what it would take to make the shift.

Francis looked around the circle and said, "This group is a good size—not too big, not too small. So let's go around and introduce ourselves. Say as little or as much as you would like about why you're here."

My heart thumped. I didn't know what to say. I didn't know why I was here, exactly, and I was also afraid of being judged. Someone volunteered to go first, a man with white hair whose wife of forty-two years had died. The person to his left was a younger man who had been in a horrible accident and struggled with chronic pain. A woman who looked seventy-something spoke of losing her home. Each person took his or her turn, like a set of tumbling dominoes. My heart thumped louder. Drug addictions, cancer, divorce, bankruptcy, discrimination. The human dominoes tumbled halfway around the circle, open, somber, yet composed.

Then it was my turn. I sat tall, my hands fidgeting in my lap, my heart thumping in my ear. "I'm here because I've had a lot of health problems." My mind was otherwise a blank. My mouth spoke as though on autopilot. "They're complex...hard to understand...hard to explain." I looked a few folks in the eye. "These problems aren't just a physical crisis, they're an existential one, too. Because, you see, I'm a doctor myself." A few folks murmured *Oh,* as I continued. "At first, I didn't believe the conditions I had were real. Even as my own body broke down, my mind was still telling me this was all in my head... Now I know differently. But I'm still trying to get to the bottom of them. My God, I *should* be better by now, it's been years... What kind of doctor am I if I can't heal myself?"

It didn't hit me until this very moment that these were my greatest shames—that I had doubted that such conditions were real until I developed them myself, and despite all I had learned and done while having the resources and time and support, I was still letting down my parents, my beloveds, the honorable name of medicine, too; and that on a beautiful Saturday, I was sitting here in a circle, admitting that I was a failure and feeling that if I had had my act together, I could have been at the zoo with my family.

When I looked up again, people were giving me gentle nods. At this wordless gesture of kindness and acceptance of my shame, I broke into tears. My hands started to tremble, and my upper body shook so hard that the chair beneath me started to shake. When I tried to talk, to contain myself, my words blurred together.

"Yes," Francis affirmed.

"I'm sorry," was all I could say.

"Please don't apologize," he said. "There's nothing as authentic as a person grieving."

"But this was supposed to be the introduction."

"There are no supposed-tos when it comes to sorrow. Our sorrow reminds us of something our ancestors knew, that our lives are intricately tied to each other, to the animals, to the plants, and to the earth. To grieve is to love."

For the rest of the morning, we did prep work—listened to poems and songs, wrote reflections in our journals—for what was to come after the lunch break: the actual ritual.

The meeting room had been rearranged during lunch. The chairs were now pushed against the walls, the photos and flowers reassembled as an altar at the front of the room. Next to the altar were baskets of smooth, black stones that Francis and the co-leader had collected from the beach that morning. He explained how the ritual would work. We would stand as a group at the back of the room, waiting until one or two or however many of us felt ready to face our grief at the altar. Others would follow a few feet behind, so we wouldn't feel alone or abandoned. At the altar, we were to hold a couple of stones, and if any tears arose, to allow them to fall onto the stones. "Now," Francis said, "we've come to the hard work of grieving."

He must have played his hand drum for ten or fifteen minutes before the first person walked up, followed by someone a few feet behind.

I watched others close their eyes and sway to the rhythms, noticing the resistance within me. To relax my body was hard. To open my soul was scary. I felt like I was clutching onto a riverbank, lest the swift current of soul take me where *it* wanted to go, rather than where *I* wanted to go. It kept tugging at me. *Let go.* Then swifter. *Let go.* Then a waterfall. *Let go!*

I closed my eyes and tried to block out any interferences in the room, allowing the vibrations of the drum to move through me, imagining it like electricity, similar to the sensations of qi during sound healing. My body began to sway. Minutes later, the floor seemed to crack open, and the ceiling fall away. The river had turned into a vast sea, and I felt myself sitting atop a fragment of ice, floating toward the edges of the earth. When I opened my eyes, I was moving toward the altar.

I located a floor pillow and sat in front of my white tapered candle. A woman to my left was wailing. I scanned the photos of strangers and pets, and the cut flowers in pretty vases. In the eyes of these dead, in the flowers that would soon be dead, too, I saw my own grief. One hand rubbing the front of my neck at the level of my thyroid, the other hand clutching two black stones, I felt the river of grief wash through me. I cried for the parts of me that had died. For the agonizing corkscrew of healing. For the dismissal by my own tribe of doctors. For the years I lost. For the life I expected but didn't get. For the losses to my children and husband, what they expected but didn't get. For the hard life lessons, one after another. Endless, they seemed.

My cries turned into sobs.

For my fear of hell, of eternal damnation. For the orchid child self I hadn't loved or accepted. For my parents, the violence they fled as children, their hardships as immigrants, the tears they were never allowed to shed. For my mother, how she met me when I needed her to, despite her own sacrifices that never came to fruition. For the violent death of Kurt, and the life he never lived. For the violence in the world, the corruption, the millions who suffered, those who didn't have access to what I had—healthy food, time for self-care, money for treatments like acupuncture, doctors or family who believed them—the disparities between those who have and those who have not. For the doctors, too, who suffered, those who carried the grief of their patients but weren't allowed to share it, those who wanted to help but didn't have the tools, those who couldn't see the grief they unknowingly caused their patients, because perhaps they had their own unseen grief. For the declining natural world. And for the absence of pause for the small things, the delicate things, the beautiful things, the slow things, the things that decayed, and what were these but the things that truly mattered, the things I truly loved.

At some point, my tears stopped, and I felt within me a thawing out, perhaps that of the frozen terror that had set in early, in my young self. I placed the stones, warm and damp in my hands, atop the other stones in the basin of water, then returned to the larger group. When the last griever finished, we gathered once again in a circle, this time standing. The same people who had tumbled like dominoes around the introductory circle now stood taller, their faces flushed, expressions changed. Francis lifted the bowl of stones, reminding us that he would return them to their original beach. There, the sea would wash our tears and absorb them into her infinite mass.

It rained hard that evening. I spent an hour in my perch, holding Rosa, then Sonia, whoever wanted to trace the crystal raindrops with me, or cast the warm breath of our lungs onto the glass. I felt a tremendous lightness of being, yet I knew there was something else I had to do.

I went to the linen closet and pulled down the shoebox with Kurt's letters. The handwritten letters were stacked in a neat pile and tied together with twine. Scattered around them were ID cards, bottle caps of his favorite beers, and ticket stubs to the Dallas rodeo, the county fair, and Texas Rangers baseball games. In a separate white envelope was the engagement ring. I fondled it with my fingers, until the rain lightened to a drizzle.

I brought the box to the back deck, and called David over.

"What's all this?" He looked at the shoebox, the matches in my hand, and the metal wastebasket. "No, sweetheart, you can't do this."

"This is the last thing I need to release."

"But you can't. This is all you have left of him."

"But healing isn't about fighting or holding on. It's about living my life, and letting go of what I need to let go of."

My hands shook as we waited for the drizzle to stop. They shook as I placed the box in the wastebasket. They shook as I struck the match. David moved behind me and held my waist. We watched the twine around the letters begin to smoke, the fibers fraying as they turned from brown to black. Within seconds of a gentle breeze rousing an orange flame, the letters caught fire, the ID cards began to melt, and the ticket stubs curled and withered. The heat grew scalding, so I took a step back, and watched the white smoke draw corkscrews in the air. Everything turned to brittle ash.

When I looked down, my hands were no longer shaking.

The week after the ritual, I felt altered. Stoned, almost. The effects were beyond mental. They were visceral.

I needed to integrate my experience. So I sought out a sanctuary. I drove around the neighborhood, coming to the first empty church I found, to see if the space felt right. No. I tried another church a few blocks down. Not the right space either. A couple of blocks farther was an Episcopal church called All Souls. The door to the sanctuary was locked, but a groundskeeper said the chapel might be open. It was a small room tucked into the underside of the building, of concrete and wooden beams, refreshingly unadorned and quaint. There were some thirty chairs packed in, a stained-glass portrait of the nativity scene, and an altar. I sat in a chair in the back, and found myself gazing upon a small crucifix in the far corner.

Instead of seeing my brokenness, as I always had before in crucifixes, I saw the outstretched arms of a God-man who embodied patient love. Patient, as in uncomplaining. Patient, as in *Love endures all things.*

Patient, as in waiting forty-plus years for me to come around to seeing that love wasn't the opposite of suffering, but was *in* suffering the same way suffering was in love. Patient, as in all the times I had died and been reborn. This patient love was common to all beings, just as qi was common to all beings, flowing within and without, everywhere. And just as we contained micro-ecosystems within us, the macro-ecosystems likewise contained us, and in fact, all the ecosystems, micro and macro, fed into each other, which meant that we contained the universe within us. This totality of All That Is, if personified, if given a name, might be called God. As I understood it now, God wasn't a fixed deity, but a living, dynamic force, an ever-unfolding continuum of All That Is. The wildest part was that *I* was an integral part of All That Is. Could it be that it wasn't about being Number One or Number Two, but simply: One? That we were all connected to everyone and everything, all integral *n*'s?

I clasped my hands, lowered my head, and whispered, "Dear God." It felt at once foreign and second-nature. No other words would come. They didn't have to. In this mysterious in-between space, I felt no fatigue or pain. There were no sounds or lights, or smells, either. No words or forms. It was the blackest black, like tar, so black it was almost purple. All the stories I had told myself vanished, and I understood not with my mind, but in my body, how love was at the root of healing. Healing seemed to be less about fighting than letting go. Here in this space, I experienced no fear. I had let go of fear!

13. Survive love and loss.

TWENTY FOUR

2019

Now, as I write in my new perch, at a corner desk in the attic facing south, I ask, Where am I today? I'm still taking care of my sensitive body. Still sticking to a nutrient-dense, whole-foods, gluten-free diet. Still practicing qigong once a day, sometimes twice, but less for specific health reasons and more because it enlivens me. Still walking five or six days a week, but resting if I need to. Still taking my vitamins, but using intuition to guide me. Still nudging my limitations, especially around driving and traveling, but living more in the present instead of worrying about the future. Still trying to keep up with an active husband—whose latest diversions include mead-making and wild boar hunting, the respective fermenting and butchering of which are performed in our kitchen, often with friends, and lots of them—but reminding myself that he, too, is mortal. Still doing occasional supportive therapies, and trying new ones like cranial osteopathy and lymphatic drainage massage. Still investigating hidden root causes if I have setbacks or hit a plateau, and reaching out to my network of colleagues for guidance. Still striving for more resilience, but not fearing setbacks or screwups or not-enoughs. And still doing deep inner work.

This certainly wasn't what I had imagined when I set off on my experiment ten years ago. But my hypothesis proved true:

I'm off the couch. *Way off.* I'm hardly on it at all.

When people ask how I am, I don't use the functionality scale anymore. There's too much change it doesn't capture. It doesn't capture the essentials like joy and hope and love—the rich hues and textures now returned in their fullness. It doesn't capture the inner freedom I experience, knowing now that I am not my illness, even during the stretches when my measurable tasks stay at the same level or dip to a lower one. Just last fall, the inflammation inside me roared up, from some new combination of the Five Causes and the Seven Essentials; and while I might have measured a 2–3 on the scale, I was surrounded by my beloveds and carried to that place of fearlessness by my inner sun, and in those regards, I felt like I was at a 10. Life can be good and hard *at the same time.*

Autoimmunity changes swiftly because life does. Rosa is now thirteen, and Sonia ten, both sharp, beautiful, strong in their sense of themselves, and different every day. My parents, after twenty years of living in Beijing, now live up the hill from us, a change of 5,900 miles. A chocolate labradoodle named Pepper also joined our family.

Pia recently got very sick. During her illness, I had the chance to use my medical and intuitive skills to help decipher why her pneumonia wasn't responding to treatment and whether her pain control was adequate. After six grueling weeks in the intensive care unit, she died. In my grief, life presented me with two new mentors: Michael Lerner, a pioneer in the integrative health field, and Rachel Remen, a leader in soul-centered medicine. They both continue to impart their wisdom and friendship. Martine Bloquiaux, the gifted intuitive, continues to teach me, as do Bob Levine and Yeshi Neumann. Together, this extraordinary team eased my return to clinical practice.

In the weeks before I returned to work, I was so hesitant. Five years was a long time to be out of practice, and applying functional medicine and intuition to patient care was uncharted territory for me. I knew, for my health's sake, I had to guard my boundaries. So I started my practice small, building it out one patient at a time, focusing largely on those with conditions similar to mine. My commute was a short and walkable distance to a one-room clinic. My hours were flexible, to accommodate David's demanding schedule, the girls, and my health.

Reinstated as "Dr. Li," I grappled with the question of whether to wear my white coat. I was aware how people might perceive the title and the name elegantly embroidered next to the lapel. But for me, none of this held the same esteem or authority anymore. It struck me as ironic—humorous, actually—that I had trained in the halls of medicine for seven grueling years and, after health challenges broke me down, had started anew, poring through years of cutting-edge science…only to return to the ancient ways of holistic thinking, intuition, mind-body integration, and ancestral diets, practices often deemed too time-consuming to be useful and not scientific enough to be valid; to say nothing of the common-sense measures of better sleep, body awareness, time in nature, detoxification, movement, nourishment, pleasure, and grief work.

In the end, I wear my white coat on some days, and my patients call me "Dr. Li." Other days, when I don't wear it, my patients, interestingly, call me "Cynthia."

I am both. I am neither.

One of my earliest patients was "Howard." His file revealed him to have a multitude of diagnoses common to "difficult patients," including irritable bowel syndrome, chronic sinusitis, anxiety disorder, depressive disorder, sleep disturbances, rosacea, and early diabetes controlled by diet. He had seen more than twenty doctors, had undergone colonoscopies, upper endoscopies, blood tests, stool tests, urine tests, and sleep studies, and was taking six to eight medications on any given day. He had been trying to watch the sugar in his diet, but he was having a tough time.

Thirty minutes before his appointment, while I was reviewing his intake forms, my focus wasn't on naming ("*What* is wrong with you?"), but on digging deeper ("*Why* are you not well?") and investigating the Five Causes of Disease, or any deficiencies of the Seven Essential Ingredients of Optimal Health.

Ten minutes before the appointment, I sat in meditation. I cleared my mind, then tried a visualization, to see if anything came up about Howard. Bringing intuition into an official clinic visit felt strange at first, but the more I would practice, the more natural it became. Breathe in, breathe out. No images came. In, out. Nothing. I continued focusing on my breath and just being present.

A young man of medium build entered, wearing a T-shirt, jeans, and an earring on the left. His demeanor was gentle, but he didn't smile. I greeted him, offered him a cup of tea, and got started.

"What are your primary hopes for your health?" I said.

One, to have more energy.

Two, to eat without worry.

Three, to clear up his skin.

I noted them in his chart, then began asking questions, populating a timeline with his family history, birth history, childhood traumas, diet history, stress levels, living and working environments, and relationships. From time to time, he ran his fingers through his dark curls, as though to ease some tension.

"This is your history," I said, showing him his timeline. "The accumulation of these small and not-so-small things, together with your genetic predispositions, produces the conditions you have."

"Painful," he said. His head and shoulders dropped.

"There's another story here, though. By introducing some small and not-so-small interventions, you can begin your healing journey."

His head and shoulders remained low. I left some space, to see what he might say. But he remained silent.

"So…" I said. Unsure where to direct the exam, I drew from my own experience with fatigue. "Are there times of day when you feel more tired?"

His head lifted. "I tend to feel lousier in the morning and late afternoon."

"I understand by looking at your timeline that you got sick a lot as a child, but was there a distinct time after which you were never the same?"

"Yes." He sat taller, looking at me as though I was clairvoyant. "I took a trip to Europe when I was in college and got food poisoning or a parasite or something, and my energy, my skin, my moods…nothing was the same after that."

On the exam table, his temperature was 97.3°F. *Suboptimal*, I mentally noted. His sweatshirt indicated he might be cold, but the day was warm. *Consider thyroid, adrenals (hormonal axis), mitochondrial dysfunction.* Resting heart rate 78. *Slightly elevated, consider deconditioning or dysautonomia.* Blood pressure 124/80. *Normal.* I noted dark circles under his eyes. *Food allergies, poor sleep, toxicity.* His face looked thin. *Chronic stress state, protein loss.* Faint acne marked his forehead. *Allergies, gut inflammation, selenium deficiency, refined sugar.* The back of his neck had marks of darker pigmentation. *Poor sugar metabolism, insulin resistance.* His tongue was cracked. *Deficiency of B vitamins.* His abdomen was slightly distended, nontender to palpation, normal liver and spleen size. *Gas trapping, gut flora imbalances, poor digestion and assimilation.* Abdominal fat. *Insulin resistance, general inflammation.* His fingernails were thin, some marked with white spots. *Zinc deficiency, essential fatty acid imbalances.* His hair, too, looked brittle. *Thyroid, protein deficiency, antioxidant deficiency.* His cardiovascular, respiratory, and neurological exams were generally unremarkable.

We sat back down at my desk. I sketched out a simple Venn diagram of three circles: genes, environment, and immune function/gut health. I explained how his gut and immune system were intricately linked, and how they affected his overall health. By the end, the paper looked like a complex subway map. Howard's eyes seemed to project both hope and fear.

I wished I could have offered him a simple answer. Like the Aha! moment in a mystery novel when the detective says "It was Mr. Jones in the lavatory with the pistol!" Years later, after seeing many more patients, I would learn that, every once in a while, a single culprit would be the case. A teenager whose attention-deficit/hyperactivity disorder (ADHD) and fatigue and hives resolved solely with the removal of gluten. Or a young mother whose migraines and premenstrual cramps and weight gain improved solely by addressing her estrogen levels. The vast majority of the time, there were multiple factors, multiple layers.

So to Howard, I said, "I know it's a lot. But if we can address the root issues, a lot of your conditions, which might seem unrelated, might heal in concert. For example, it's possible you're deficient in magnesium. This can contribute to the diabetes, the insomnia, the mood swings, as well as the digestive symptoms. What I'm trying to say is, we've got a lot to work with."

He wanted to know how long it would be before he saw results. Again, I wished for a more definitive answer. The most accurate answer: "It depends." It depended on his stress levels. How quickly he could implement the dietary changes. How much support he had. Whether or not he could fit in exercise or a mind-body practice. What root causes or deficiencies we could identify and treat.

"You're the captain of this ship," I told him. Whether the journey was choppy or smooth, I was his navigator. He probably wasn't used to this kind of doctor-patient relationship. I wasn't either.

When we got to the treatment plan, I knew he didn't have much money to spend on specialty tests or alternative therapies like acupuncture or massage. So I kept his prescription for the first phase of his healing as simple and low-cost as possible: a thirty-day anti-inflammatory diet (frozen foods if fresh was too expensive); probiotic foods; digestive enzymes; a multivitamin with a good proportion of key vitamins and minerals, and extra doses of magnesium and vitamin D. As he left, I gave him a lab slip to screen for nutrient deficiencies, celiac disease, various markers of inflammation, sugar metabolism, and a purge stool sample to screen for stealth gut infections. I also tore a handwritten sheet off my prescription pad.

"Here are your other prescriptions. Aim for twice a day, with or without food."

The prescription said:

1.   Walk in nature, 15 minutes, 5 times a week, barefoot if possible.

2.   Practice pleasure. If nothing gives you pleasure, watch funny videos and make sure you're laughing. Genuine or fake, it doesn't matter.

3.   Look in the mirror and say, "I am whole." Repeat 10 times. Best done naked.

He read the paper and laughed.

"They're harder than they look," I said, giving him a smile. "Because they ask you to pay attention to yourself. That's the only way you can heal."

After he left, I typed up my doctor's note. Then I closed my laptop, drank some water, and spent another ten minutes in meditation, clearing myself of the encounter with Howard and preparing for the next patient. I was ready to open my eyes, when an image popped up: a small pouch. The appendix? No. The cecum? No. The gall bladder? *Yes*. Was this a clue that the next patient had chronic digestive issues, or gall-stones, or an infection? Tapping into my intuition felt like accessing a database of infinite knowledge that could help narrow things down with greater precision. It almost felt like cheating.

Charged up, I opened the electronic chart and combed her questionnaires page by page, having a very good time.

14. Reclaim your purpose.

A couple of months before my "coming out" presentation to main-stream medicine at Grand Rounds, I contemplated how to get my broader message across. I pulled out my file of "keepers," articles in medicine worth holding onto, and got sidetracked by a famous essay called "Arrogance," published in the prestigious *New England Journal of Medicine* in 1980. It was a piece my beloved mentor, Dr. Eisenberg, had given me when I was just starting out in my clinical rotations.

Franz Ingelfinger, a former editor of the journal, had written the essay as he lay dying. He was highlighting a lack of empathy in the profession at the time and posing a singular question: How different would medicine be if medical schools only admitted students who had themselves experienced a serious illness?

Something within me stirred. Sure, doctors could use more empathy, and sure, most of us learn best through personal experience. But the present-day health-care crisis felt different. I didn't agree that most doctors were inherently arrogant or brusque. The curt bedside manner and severed doctor-patient relationships were largely symptoms of burnout from a broken system.

The statistics were growing dire. In one survey of five thousand doctors across specialties, a clear majority wouldn't advise a young person to go into medicine. In another survey, close to half reported feeling detached or unfulfilled. Suicide and depression rates were higher among doctors than in many other professions. Increasingly, doctors in practice wanted to leave their careers behind. Perhaps it was the appointment times that were impossibly short; or the lack of general support; or the lack of more satisfying treatment options for chronic ailments; or the mounting busyness of emails, phone calls, insurance schemes, and electronic medical records… Most likely, it was multiple factors interacting synergistically, as in the Ecological Paradigm of Health, *squeezing, squeezing,* and making doctors feel like powerless Number Twos to the Healthcare Giant.

The thought of more doctors falling ill as I had, waiting for change to happen, felt cruel and unimaginable. Besides, there were millions of patients suffering *now,* those we had gone into medicine to serve. Returning to my presentation, I knew I wanted to offer something beyond a new paradigm of medicine. I wanted to offer an ounce of hope with regard to the system. But how could I convey hope if I was feeling overwhelmed by the size of the problem?

That night, David was changing out of his clothes, and threw his GET SOME SUN T-shirt onto the floor. He had ten or fifteen of these same shirts from his first solar campaign.

David! I thought. He was a big-picture thinker. He had long worked on systemic change. He had been addressing an existential threat of another kind to our common humanity.

I told him how I was struggling. "The problems feel so huge, I don't even know where to start," I sighed.

"Ok, so the medical system is sick."

"Yes!" I said, seeing his point.

"What would you prescribe for your sick patient?"

I took Ingelfinger's idea, but held in mind a different singular question: How different would medicine be if the requisite wasn't a serious illness, but instead was an immersion in wellness? I reviewed in my mind the Seven Essential Ingredients of Optimal Health, and my new learner's mind spouted off a list:

More permission for doctors to say "I don't know." Or, for that matter, to say "No," and set clear boundaries for themselves.

Permission for doctors to get more sleep.

And to have more gardens, arboretums, and houseplants in medical facilities.

And to use safer chemicals inside.

And to develop their intuition.

And to choose whole foods in hospitals and nursing homes.

And to play.

And to grieve.

Above all, permission to eradicate from medical culture the implicit motto, *What doesn't kill you makes you stronger.* Because it *was* killing us.

"It sounds so idealistic," I said to David. "And what about the underserved communities, those who are most vulnerable to nutrient deficiencies, pollution, and social stresses?" I flopped onto the bed. "I'm just an *n* of 1—a diminished *n*, at that."

"Change has to start somewhere, right?"

David was right. I might be an *n* of 1, I thought, but I was an integral *n* to All That Is. I didn't have to change the world. I just needed to take the next step.

A few weeks later, twenty doctors and I were sitting in a circle around our living room. Several integrative-functional medicine doctors, a few pediatricians and family practitioners, an obstetrician-gynecologist, a couple of ER doctors, and a few retirees looking for the "next gig." Martine, my intuition mentor, was present, too. I had sent out emails to invite doctors who might be interested in exploring integrative principles, as well as intuition. The topics were broad. This was merely a gathering to explore the topics. To start a conversation.

We talked about the wellness programs already implemented in their various clinical settings. Then how to expand them. There were also wellness programs underway in internships and residencies. At once, I felt heartened about what existed and impatient for the magnitude that was still needed.

In the second half, Martine reviewed some basic principles of intuition and shared a story of how she felt signals in her body. Others shared stories, starting out vague, like "I had a hunch there was something wrong with my patient." But before long, we started going deeper. I shared how I used intuition to hone in on medications or supplements. Then a family practitioner shared how he connected energetically with a baby he was soon to deliver from a high-risk patient, saying, "I just knew the baby would die if I didn't intervene."

There was a pause. We were checking each other out for reactions. When no one scoffed, all sorts of stories emerged. Someone shared a story of how she came up with an unlikely diagnosis of "neurocysticercosis," a parasite in the brain that wasn't common in the States, for the cause of her patient's headaches. "I literally saw an image of the worm's head when I looked at the patient." She raised an eyebrow, seemingly still in disbelief about it. "Okay," she mumbled, as though to herself, "that was the first time I've ever said that out loud, and it feels kinda weird."

The workshop lasted all day Saturday, and concluded Sunday morning. It felt part grief ritual—confessing secret stories and releasing the shame we harbored—and part initiation—a rite into a quietly subversive movement. We were recognizing each other as fellow sojourners upholding the tenets of our profession but expanding the spaces in between, following in the footsteps of all the healers who had come before us.

I knew I wouldn't be alone during my Grand Rounds talk the following week.

After everyone left, I cleaned up, reorganized the chairs, and checked my watch: a quarter to 1 p.m. Time to roll out the television cart. Like clockwork, David, the girls, and Pepper returned from their swim and hike in Strawberry Canyon. I asked the girls to give Pepper a rinse, then shower themselves off, and hang their towels out to dry. David was in the kitchen, popping some popcorn. At 12:55, he moved to the living room. The 49ers game was about to start. Contented, I sat in my perch, opened my journal, and jotted some reflections of the intuition circle.

With my beloveds each ensconced in their busyness, I continued, pen to paper, wanting to write more than mere mental notes. I used to write in my journal all the time—stories from the day, reflections of the past, poems, songs. *It started as a flutter,* I wrote. Then, *It felt like a baby chick ruffling its feathers beneath my breastbone.* I looked at the weeping cypress, remembering the darker moments—the undertow, the vertigo, the labor contractions—and then, *pop-pop-pop.*

I wrote until halftime. The 49ers were up by three, David cheered. The sun was high above the Golden Gate.

And I was *here.*

15. Find your story, the real one.

How to Get Off the Couch
(a.k.a. How to Heal)

1. Ask new questions.

2. Reset your inner clock.

3. Give yourself permission to receive.

4. Get a daily dose of nature.

5. Detoxify the house (and yourself).

6. Let intuition tell your thinking mind where to look next.

7. Change your thoughts, change your genes.

8. Inhabit your body.

9. Heal the gut.

10. Break old habits that no longer serve you.

11. Practice pleasure. It's serious work.

12. Investigate hidden root causes.

13. Survive love and loss.

14. Reclaim your purpose.

15. Find your story, the real one.

Part Three

How to Heal

More than a set of actions, healing is a state of being. It requires a shift in mindset, a reorientation toward the mind, body, and spirit. That said, a guideline of actions to follow, if practiced regularly, can open you to this new state of being, transforming your relationship to yourself and your environment.

The journey of healing is *deep*. It goes down to the root causes and addresses the mechanisms of disease.

It is *slow*. It honors the pace of nature.

If you're like me, you would prefer healing to be less deep and less slow. But healing is the corkscrew path of the human condition—it spans the lowest lows and the highest highs. If, on your journey, you feel like you're back to square one, remember the spiral: you might in fact be at a different level.

In the following pages are some suggestions I give to my patients. I have either tried or adopted these practices myself. Some are widely accessible and low- or no-cost. Others, less so. The greatest resource they demand, as a whole, is your attention. They are "practices," meaning they take time and commitment to develop. They ask you to pause, and break from the conveniences of modern life. You don't have to do all of them at once; in fact, I discourage my patients from doing so. The important thing is to tune in to your body's needs, put forth your best effort, and fold the practices into your life.

What you do now can impact your health for years to come. And if you're of childbearing age or younger, your changes may benefit the health of your future children, too.

These guidelines are less a goal of self-improvement than a gradual initiation into caring for the one body you've been given in this lifetime.

So go slow, go deep.

1. Ask new questions.

This is no small task. It's especially challenging for doctors, scientists, academics, or others steeped in the belief that we can "fix whatever's broke" or think our way out of an unfortunate situation. Symptoms are our bodies' way of saying something isn't working anymore. Often, these symptoms have been going on for a while, but we've dismissed or overridden them with mind-over-matter techniques.

Now it's time to pay attention and suspend disbelief. The rational mind allows us to make sense of our discoveries, but it's our leaps in consciousness that drive discovery.

2. Reset your inner clock.

To be healthy is to be in sync with your inner and outer rhythms. Your organs have their own circadian rhythms, turning on and off at different times in a twenty-four-hour cycle, and your days are governed by the rhythms of sunlight, among other forces.

Eating: The more regular, the better. A regular schedule allows your digestive organs and all the hormones involved in digesting, absorbing, and using food for energy, to function optimally. Having a twelve- to fourteen-hour window of fasting overnight is also ideal for most. If you have chronic fatigue, you may need to eat more often.

Suggested meal sizes: a big breakfast, medium-size lunch, and small dinner.

Suggested eating window: 8 a.m. to 8 p.m. If you're able, 8 a.m. to 6 p.m. (But if you have chronic fatigue or dysautonomia symptoms, you may need a longer eating window, like 8 a.m. to 9 or 10 p.m.)

Sleeping: Consistent sleep is necessary for energy and mental focus, as well as for detoxification, tissue growth, and repair. According to the Centers for Disease Control, more than 35 percent of American adults don't get the recommended seven hours a night.

Restful sleep is enhanced by nighttime rituals, but studies also reveal the importance of daytime states. Decreasing chronic stress during wakefulness enhances sleep quality and duration.

For those with chronic sleep disorders, seek proper guidance from a health care professional to correct physiological imbalances.

Suggestions:

1. Rise with clarity in the morning.

    *   Get up at roughly the same time every day (and go to bed around the same time).

    *   Get at least 20 minutes of bright light exposure after waking.

2. Regulate activity and rest.

    *   Brisk exercise or a meditation routine are great ways to start the day.

    *   If your job requires prolonged sitting, set a timer so that every hour, you get up and stretch and walk around.

    *   Do simple stress-relieving meditations throughout the day (see **6. Let intuition tell your thinking mind where to look next** for examples).

3. Prepare for sleep.

    *   Avoid strenuous exercise at least 2–3 hours before bedtime.

    *   Avoid caffeine or sugary foods, especially in the evenings.

    *   Check medications for sleep-disrupting side effects and talk to your doctor about alternatives.

    *   Limit alcohol intake. Drinking less, earlier, and with food is best.

4. Follow the rhythm of the sun.

    *   At dusk, dim the lights.

    *   Reduce exposure to blue light by turning off laptops and cell phones; or download and/or activate blue light filter programs on your electronic devices.

    *   Develop a soothing ritual after dusk to ready your mind and body for sleep: a warm bath, journal writing, a good book, a massage, or intimacy.

5. Create a sleep sanctuary.

    •   Keep the bedroom cool (65 degrees or less).

    •   Move clocks out of sight (they pull us back into wakefulness).

    •   Remove electronic devices (cell phones, tablets, laptops) from the bedroom.

    •   Sleep in darkness. Use blackout curtains or eyeshades.

    •   Keep the bed sacred, only for sleep or sex.

    •   Don't just "go to sleep." Practice letting go of wakefulness.

6. Tune in to your body.

    •   Go to bed when you feel sleepy.

    •   If you can't sleep, get up and relax in a comfortable place until you feel sleepy.

    •   Avoid stimulating activities. If your mind is racing with to-dos, jot them down and tell your mind you don't have to keep track of them right now.

My favorite sleep aids[*]:

•   Magnesium, chelated forms. Glycinate is my favorite. If you're prone to constipation, citrate is a good form. 400–600 mg at bedtime, avoid if you have a history of kidney disease.

•   5-HTP, an amino acid that helps your body make more melatonin. Starting dose of 100 mg at bedtime.

•   Melatonin, liposomal or time-released formulas. Starting dose of 0.5 mg, and titrated up, if necessary, to 1–2 mg. If higher doses are required, see a health care professional to rule out other causes of insomnia. Taking too much melatonin can suppress your body's own production of this hormone.

---

[*] As with all supplements, vitamins, and medications, consult your health care practitioner if you are breastfeeding or pregnant, or if you have chronic kidney or liver disease.

Since the quality of supplements can vary, you can research common brands on **http://www.consumerlab.com** for a low-cost membership fee.

- Valerian root. 400–500 mg, 1–2 capsules before bedtime.

- Ashwagandha root. 500 mg of a capsule or tincture standardized to 2.5–5 percent with anolides, 1–2 capsules before bedtime.

Resources:

- *The Circadian Code: Lose Weight, Supercharge Your Energy, and Transform Your Health from Morning to Midnight* by Satchin Panda, PhD

- *Go to Bed!* by Sarah Ballantyne, PhD (available at www.the paleomom.com)

- *Say Good Night to Insomnia: The Six-Week, Drug-Free Program Developed at Harvard Medical School* by Gregg D. Jacobs, PhD

- Insight Timer, a free app that has more than ten thousand guided meditations. The body scans and abdominal breathing practices help bring awareness into your body.

3. Give yourself permission to receive.

Healing doesn't occur in isolation. The people and environment with which you surround yourself can support your journey. But first, you have to open yourself up to receive. Let go of shoulds and should-nots. And reach out.

1.   Find a practitioner you trust. Ultimately, the trust is more important than what kind of medicine or therapy s/he practices.

    a.   Functional medicine practitioners: **http://www.function almedicine.org**.

    b.   Functional medicine health coaches: **http://www.func tionalmedicinecoaches.org**.

    c.   Cranial osteopaths: **http://www.cranialacademy.org**.

    d.   Acupuncturists: **http://www.nccaom.org**.

2. Talk with your partner or a close friend. And make sure your partner is talking with his or her close friend(s), too.

3. If your energy is low or your brain is foggy, consider setting up a rotating meal service, where friends and family can sign up to drop off food. You can specify your dietary needs and preferences. **http://www.mealtrain.com.**

4. If friends ask to help, suggest practical things: grocery shopping, laundry, medication/supplement pick-up, whatever is most helpful to you.

5. Connect with a support group for chronic fatigue patients and caregivers, by phone or in person. Try AMMES (American Myalgic Encephalomyelitis and Chronic Fatigue Syndrome Society): **http://www.ammes.org.**

4. Get a daily dose of nature.

If getting outside is logistically challenging, bring in houseplants or fresh flowers. Any bit of nature can stimulate the healing rest-and-digest phase.

If your system is sensitive to plants and flowers, consider images of calming nature scenes.

If you're bed- or housebound, make a point to spend your days in a light-filled room. Try to get out to your deck or into your yard for part of the day, too.

5. Detoxify the house (and yourself).

Here are some ways to clean up your home environment. Consider making these changes slowly but surely rather than all at once, so as not to overwhelm yourself or your family.

1. Choose organic produce and meats whenever possible. (See the resources below for prioritizing produce.)

2. Shop at a farmer's market if available.

3. Use stainless steel and/or ceramic cookware. Avoid non-stick pots and pans.

4. For food storage, use Pyrex glass containers or recycled jars. Avoid storing or heating food in any type of plastic container. Also, choose beverages in glass bottles over aluminum cans when available.

5. Filter chlorine from your drinking water, as well as other chemicals and pollutants. For good-quality basic water filters, go to www.multipure.com.

6. Use an air purifier in your home and office to reduce allergens.

7. Remove dust by using a vacuum cleaner with a HEPA filter, and vacuum often. Avoid sweeping as a regular way to remove dust, as this can aerosolize mold and other dust, which may carry pollutants.

8. Wash hands with warm water and castile soap. Avoid artificial fragrances, antibacterial soaps, and harsh astringents.

9. Use biodegradable cleaning products or diluted vinegar or hydrogen peroxide for cleaning and disinfecting. Avoid chlorine bleach.

10. Reduce/eliminate plastics that off-gas. Anything that smells "chemical," like vinyl shower curtains and synthetic carpets and padding.

11. Use paints and other solvents that are low- or no-VOC (volatile organic compound) products.

12. Choose personal care products with essential oils over synthetic fragrances.

13. Choose couches that aren't sprayed with flame retardants.

14. Reduce electro-pollution from EMF. Put your Wi-Fi modem on an overnight timer so it automatically shuts off during sleeping hours. Remove electric appliances that are close to the bed.

Never wear your cell phone on your body. Keep your phone in airplane mode when not in use.

15. Go beyond your own home. Support policies that promote cleaner alternatives. A healthier planet depends on healthier personal choices, and healthier individuals depend on a healthier planet.

My favorite resources:

- **http://www.ewg.org**. Wondering which foods to buy organic? Which personal health-care products are healthier? Which safer insect repellants actually work? Environmental Working Group is a nonprofit advocacy group with practical guidelines for everyday living.

- **http://www.becausehealth.org**. An at-a-glance compilation of science-based tips, guides, and expert advice to create a healthier future for you and your communities.

- **http://www.healthandenvironment.org**. Wondering how to get involved at the community level and beyond? Shifting the responsibility onto governmental agencies and industries reduces the responsibility from the individual or family. Collaborative on Health and the Environment is an international association of scientists, health professionals, activists, policy-makers, and community folks working together to review the latest science.

- **http://www.nrdc.org**. National Resources Defense Council is an environmental action group focused on a variety of environmental policies.

- **http://www.epa.org**. The US Environmental Protection Agency has a comprehensive pollutants database.

- For more resources, see: **http://www.cynthialimd.com /environmental-health-resources.**

Here are a few tips to clean up the inner environment of your body. Because you are what you eat, drink, breathe, touch, and that which you cannot eliminate.

Detox basics. When I use the term "detox," I'm not referring to high-end spas or extreme juicing fasts, which can strain your budget and harm your body. Detoxification is simply the body's innate capacity to filter and eliminate unwanted substances that would otherwise build up and contribute to chronic disease. Several organs assist us with this process (the skin, gut, immune system, lungs, and kidneys), although the primary organ is the liver.

The deeper story. Your individual capacity to detoxify depends on multiple factors: (1) your genes, (2) your cumulative exposure to environmental pollutants, (3) the health of your gut, (4) regular elimination by the gut (stool) and kidneys (urine), (5) the availability of key nutrients for the liver, and (6) your age.

What to remove (or reduce)?

1. Personal exposures through more informed choices (per above).

2. Overall environmental exposures in your communities, by advocating for industries to use safer alternatives (see resources below).

What to restore? Your body's innate detox processes.

Here are 10 steps to do so:

1. Do a lemon juice cleanse. First thing in the morning, before you eat or drink anything (before any medicines or supplements), squeeze the juice of one fresh lemon, dilute with room-temperature, filtered water to your preference, and drink. Wait 20 minutes before eating or drinking anything else. Do this daily for 3–4 weeks.

2. Eat your broccoli. Compounds in the Brassica family—kale, collards, beets, cauliflower, cabbage—boost your liver's detox enzymes, while providing other nutrients and antioxidants.

Steam them, boil them, or mix them into a smoothie. See **9. Heal the gut** for specifics on a detox diet.

3. Remember your protein. Amino acids like glycine boost your liver's detox enzymes, and cysteine is a necessary cofactor for the proteins that detoxify heavy metals. Bone broth, beans, and wild, oily fish are good sources.

4. Increase your fiber. Aim for regular bowel movements, 1–2 times a day. Good sources of fiber: non-starchy vegetables, nuts, seeds, flaxseed meal, and beans. Fiber supplements like psyllium or rice bran are alternative choices (~30 g per day + plenty of water), as are prebiotic supplements (different than probiotics, these are the fibers that feed healthy gut flora).

5. Get sweaty. Exercise and take some saunas. Sweat can carry out everyday chemicals like phthalates and PCBs (perfluorinated compounds). After sweating, shower off with castile soap, like Dr. Bronner's, so the chemicals don't get reabsorbed into your body.

6. Eat the foods that bind. Certain foods naturally bind heavy metals and remove them from our bodies. These include cilantro, apples, pears, citrus (especially the rinds, if grated and used in salad dressings), carrots, and beets. Sulfur-containing vegetables like onions, leeks, garlic, and asparagus support the detox of heavy metals like lead, cadmium, and mercury.

7. Go coconuts. Coconut water can hydrate you like IV fluids. A liter of this electrolyte-rich beverage daily during detox periods, along with 6–8 cups of water, can help your kidney systems flush out the waste.

8. Share a cup of tea. A compound in green tea (EGCG) can boost liver enzymes and also provide antioxidants. Opt for decaffeinated green tea if you're sensitive to caffeine or have sleep difficulties. Or brew yourself a cup of turmeric tea. One of my favorite teas is a dropper full of Swedish bitters (a combination of detox herbs, including turmeric and milk thistle) with hot water.

9. Include magnesium. This mighty mineral is involved in hundreds of important chemical reactions in the body, many of which are involved in detoxification. Supplement with a form that is well-absorbed, like glycinate or malate or citrate, and aim for 400–600 mg a day (note: this is not for those with underlying kidney disease). Soaking in a bath of Epsom salts can also provide a small dose.

10. Get your ha-has. Laughter boosts circulation, gets digestion moving along, and improves sleep. Laugh while doing numbers 1–9 above! (If you have to, fake it till you feel it.)

My favorite supplements to aid detox:

- Magnesium, as detailed above

- A good B-complex with active folate (5-MTHF or 5-methylfolate), starting with 400–800 mg daily

- Curcumin (turmeric extract, in the absorbable form of Meriva), 500–1,000 mg twice daily

- N-acetylcysteine (NAC), 500 mg daily

- Vitamin C, buffered or ester form, 1,000 mg once or twice daily

- A multi-mineral complex with selenium, zinc, and chromium (but without iron)

My favorite detox websites:

- **http://www.drhyman.com** (10-day detox course)

- **http://www.detoxinista.com**

- **http://www.balancedbites.com** (21-day sugar detox)

6. Let intuition tell your thinking mind where to look next.

Intuition is a form of knowing that doesn't depend on scientific proof. More of an experiential resonance, intuition can be developed by tuning into sensations, images, and observation in hindsight. I see intuition as another "data set," like seeing with a second eye, telling your thinking mind where to look next—which allows us more depth and breadth of knowledge.

Here are a few simple practices you can do to develop your intuition:

1. Meditate. Finding your inner stillness is the foundation of developing intuition, because it settles the thinking mind.

    Here are two simple meditations:

    *   Simple meditation 1:

        Find a comfortable chair.

        Grab a throw blanket so you don't get cold.

        Light a candle.

        Stare at the flame while focusing on your breath. In-breath, out-breath.

        If your mind wanders, refocus on the flame and your breath.

        Think of your thoughts as clouds and let them float away.

    *   Simple meditation 2:

        Find a comfortable chair.

        Grab a throw blanket so you don't get cold.

        Pick a mantra that is relaxing to you. (Ex.: I am held, I've done enough today, It's time to rest now.)

        Consider setting a timer for 10–15 minutes, or start with shorter intervals.

        Close your eyes.

        Breathe deeply, from your abdomen, and repeat the mantra ten times.

        Repeat until your time is up.

2. Visualize. Here's a visualization practice my friend and mentor Pia taught me:

    Find a comfortable chair and sit upright.

Take 10 deep breaths, relax your shoulders, and clear your mind.

Visualize walking through a forest, or a field of cornstalks, or a lush garden.

Visualize coming to an open beach. Hold that scene in your mind's eye for as long as you can, and see what emerges. Objects or people that emerge from the left represent the past. Those from the right represent the future.

Record the images in your journal. Writing helps to consolidate the experience.

3. Do timed automatic writings to quiet your rational mind. See **13. Survive love and loss** for directions.

4. Record your dreams in a journal. Note patterns, repetitions, symbols, and archetypes, rather than literal events. Before sleep, invite your subconscious for revelation through dreams.

5. Pay attention to your body's signals: twinges, goosebumps, or nausea, for example. Intuitive signals tend to be fleeting, whereas signals that represent physical imbalances or disease tend to be longer-lasting.

6. Enlist the gift of hindsight. This can help to correlate images and signs with actual happenings, and decipher between intuition and wishful or fearful thinking. Record these notes into your dream journal, which may be used for all intuition-related reflections.

7. Be patient. Developing intuition is like learning a new language. It takes time, repetition, and practice.

8. Practice humility and trust. Like analytical thinking, intuition isn't 100 percent accurate 100 percent of the time.

My favorite resources for developing intuition:

*   *Second Sight: An Intuitive Psychiatrist Tells Her Extraordinary Story and Shows You How to Tap Your Own Inner Wisdom* by Judith Orloff, MD

- *The Intuitive Way: The Definitive Guide to Increasing Your Awareness*, a hands-on workbook by Penney Peirce

- *The ABCs of Energy: An Easy Guide to What You Feel But Can't See* by Martine Bloquiaux

7. Change your thoughts, change your genes.

What you think can turn certain genes on and others off, and change the patterns by which your neurons connect. Here are some ideas and practices that can get your brain out of the vicious fight-or-flight cycle, which generates inflammation, and into the rest-and-digest healing state.

1. Mix things up. Rearrange furniture and decor, eat with your non-dominant hand, sleep on the other side of the bed, walk or drive a new route.

2. Learn or revisit a musical instrument. This doesn't have to be a huge commitment. Borrow a ukulele or buy one for $20 and learn a few songs via YouTube.

3. Listen to music from a time in your past that was positive and life-affirming. If you can't think of such a time, listen to music that feels life-affirming to you.

4. Identify harmful thought patterns. When they arise, note them, tell them to stop, and redirect your thoughts to something positive. Some harmful patterns: obsessing about your health, trying to predict how you'll feel in certain situations, engaging in negative self-talk, self-blame, addictive behaviors, justifying negative beliefs.

5. When you catch yourself in these negative patterns, infuse your mind instead with a positive experience—this must be visualized and embodied. Here is a visualization adapted from the Dynamic Neural Retraining System by Annie Hopper:

   Think of a positive memory. Experiences in water (swimming, jumping into a lake) are especially effective for this exercise.

Describe this memory aloud in present tense and imagine it with all your senses. (What does it feel like on my skin? What does it smell like? What does it look like? What sounds do I hear?) You're going for evoked sensations, like goosebumps, a shiver, or a warm sensation in your body. Only then have you triggered the vagus nerve.

Anchor this experience with a positive mantra (ex.: I am strong!, I am healthy!, I am living my life!).

Practice this daily. Twice a day if possible. Repetition is the key to rewiring your brain.

And eliciting the visceral experiences is key to healing your body.

My favorite resources for neural retraining:

- The Dynamic Neural Retraining System by Annie Hopper. **http://www.retrainingthebrain.com.**

- *The Brain's Way of Healing: Remarkable Discoveries from the Frontiers of Neuroplasticity* by Norman Doidge, MD

- *Buddha's Brain: The Practical Neuroscience of Happiness, Love, and Wisdom* by Rick Hanson, PhD

- *Train Your Mind, Change Your Brain: How a New Science Reveals Our Extraordinary Potential to Transform Ourselves* by Sharon Begley

8. Inhabit your body.

When you start to inhabit your body after years or decades of being disconnected, your symptoms may feel more intense at first, because you're noticing more. Try not to fear the sensations—better yet, move toward them. They're merely your body's way of showing you the underlying deficiencies and imbalances.

Here are some ways to reconnect the brain and the body:

1. Stimulate the vagus. This nerve is the godfather of the rest-and-digest state of the nervous system, which reduces inflammation and promotes healing. Like any other nerve, the more you activate it, the stronger the response.

    - Get throaty. Gargle with water several times a day. This action uses muscles in the back of your throat, which stimulates the vagus. Imagine you are gargling from deep within your esophagus.

    - Belt it out. At home alone, in the shower, or in the car, sing as loudly as you can. This also uses muscles in the back of your throat.

    - Chew your food. Remove distractions like phones and screens, and pay attention to your meal. By chewing thoroughly until you fully mash the food in your mouth, you not only facilitate the digestive process, you also stimulate the vagus.

    - Gag yourself. Take a spoon with a rounded handle, or if you prefer, purchase a box of tongue blades from the pharmacy. Don't jab yourself in the back of the throat. Instead, open your mouth wide and push down on the back part of your tongue with the blade/spoon, activating the gag reflex. Repeat this several times.

    - Breathe from your belly. Sit quietly, relax your shoulders, and do 20–30 deep, slow abdominal breaths. Abdominal breathing stems from your belly, not your chest, so start by placing your hand over your belly. Feel your belly push your hand out with each inhalation. After each inhalation, hold your breath gently for five to seven seconds, then exhale slowly, using your abdominal muscles to push out as much air as you can.

    - Finish your next shower cold. Exposure to cold water can trigger the vagus nerve. Try 10 or 20 seconds of cold water. You're going for a shiver response.

2. Start your day with a shot of qi.

    - Do a 10-minute qigong practice. Many free guided practices are available on YouTube.

    - Tap your organs: chest for lungs, under the rib cage for the liver and spleen, the small of your back for the kidneys and reproductive system, the belly for the digestive system.

    - Sound healing: see the resources below for chanting practices purported to activate and strengthen internal organs.

3. Go for a swim, or take a bath. Being immersed in water is a sensory experience that can awaken the body. Add 5–10 drops of lavender essential oils for a heightened sensory experience.

4. Walk outside, barefoot. The soles of the feet have more than a hundred thousand sensory nerves that send signals to the brain. When we always wear shoes, our brain loses out on these connections with the body. A walk on the beach, among the different textures of sand and water, is an ideal place. Your backyard works, too. See **4. Get a daily dose of nature** for more details.

My favorite resources for inhabiting the body:

- **www.chicenter.com** has subscriptions for videotaped and livestream qigong practices for all levels. There are also free demonstrations by Master Mingtong Gu on YouTube.

- Four-Minute Workout by Zach Bush, MD, via YouTube; do this at your own pace and capacity.

- Fightmaster Yoga via YouTube has free yoga practices for beginners.

- Jessica Smith TV via YouTube has easy twenty- and thirty-minute stretching practices.

9. Heal the gut.

Exposing yourself to natural habitats, especially the soil, increases your exposure to diverse microorganisms that can benefit your gut ecology. So when you're practicing **4. Get a daily dose of nature**, play in the grass or the dirt. Or while taking a hike, feel the leaves of an oak or rub a fern against your cheek.

The most direct way to increase gut diversity is by *what you eat*. There are many versions of a gut-healing, energy-boosting, anti-inflammatory diet. The common features are: (1) whole foods, (2) rich in quantity and colors of vegetables, (3) low in processed starches and sugars, (4) high in healthy fats and protein, (5) high in fiber that feeds healthy gut flora, or probiotic foods that support gut flora. A short-term "reset" diet can differ from a longer-term maintenance diet, but the former is a good foundation for the latter. A common misunderstanding is that once you find a diet that heals what ails you, you stick to it forever. Remember, your body is an ecosystem. It changes with time, with circumstances. Different foods are needed for different health and disease states. And staying on too limited a diet for the longer-term may diminish the diversity of your gut flora.

Here's the 30-day diet I did.

The Basics of the 30-Day Reset Diet

This 30-day diet is designed to improve digestion, rebalance the gut flora, reduce inflammation, and identify food sensitivities and/or allergies. As a result, most people experience an increase in energy and a normalization of weight (meaning weight loss if you're over, weight gain if you're under). It addresses the two basic questions of functional medicine:

What to remove? Commonly problematic foods (allergens, processed, refined).

What to restore? Nutrient-dense foods, with an emphasis on fresh vegetables.

It's essential that you make these changes for at least 30 continuous days. If your health challenges are more chronic or complex, 45 or 60 days may be better. One "cheat" here or there may trigger new reactions, so keep this month (or two) as clean as possible.

A few basic guidelines:

- Eat at the kitchen table with no other distractions. (No electronic devices.)

- Chew your food. Don't inhale it.

- Eat 3 regular meals a day. If you have diabetes or chronic fatigue, it is better that you eat 4 smaller meals, to keep your blood sugars more stable.

- The more food you can cook, the better. The more from scratch, the better, too.

- Choose organic meats and produce whenever possible.

- Use a slow cooker to cook for you. Cook in batches. Freeze the extras.

What to restore?[**]

- All vegetables. Aim for 5–8 servings a day of a rainbow-colored assortment.

- All fruits. Aim for 3–5 servings. Favor low-sugar fruits like berries and peaches.

- All seeds.

- All nuts.

- All meats. Fresh (ex: stewed chicken) over processed (ex: sausage). Include organ meats.

- All broths.

- All eggs.

** Established food allergies must still be avoided, of course.

- All fish and shellfish. Include fatty fish like salmon (wild), mackerel, sardines.

- All unprocessed fats. Olive oil, avocado oil, ghee (clarified butter, which doesn't contain casein or other milk proteins), coconut oil, tallow, lard.

- All teas. Especially green, red (rooibos), and herbal teas. Coffee and black tea in moderation.

Include daily:

- Bone broth soups—an easy bone broth recipe: http://www .cynthialimd.com/nutrient-dense-cooking-basics/. Cook in batches, freeze the extras.

- Fermented foods—sauerkraut, pickles (naturally fermented, not made with vinegar), kimchi, kvass.

- Filtered tap water, sparkling water, and coconut water.

What to remove?

- Dairy. From cows, goats, and sheep (including butter).

- Grains. For the more intensive version of this 30-day diet, eliminate all grains. This is important for those with digestive or autoimmune conditions.

- If this feels undoable for a full month, add in a small serving a day of gluten-free grains like white rice or quinoa.

- If that still feels undoable, consider a whole-foods diet rich in vegetables that is strictly gluten- and dairy-free.

- Legumes. Beans of all kinds (soy, black, kidney, pinto, etc.), lentils, and peanuts. Green peas and snap peas are okay.

- Sweeteners, real or artificial. Sugar, high-fructose corn syrup, maple syrup, honey, agave, Splenda, Equal, NutraSweet, xylitol, stevia, etc.

- Processed or refined snack foods.

- Sodas and diet sodas.

- Alcohol in any form.

- White potatoes.

- Premade sauces and seasonings.

How to avoid common pitfalls:

- Prepare well beforehand. Choose a time frame during which you will have limited or reduced travel, and that doesn't include holidays or special occasions.

- Study the list of foods allowed on the diet and make a shopping list.

- Remove the foods from your pantry or refrigerator that aren't allowed on the diet, if that makes it easier.

- Engage the whole family to try this together, or find a friend to join you. Success happens in community.

- Set up a calendar to mark your progress. Print out a free 30-day online calendar, tape it to the refrigerator door, and mark off each day.

- Pack snacks with you, pack your lunch, call ahead to restaurants to check their menu (or check online).

- Get enough vegetables and fats.

- If you feel jittery or lose too much weight, increase your carbohydrates (starchy vegetables like yams, taro, sweet potatoes).

- Don't misread withdrawal-type symptoms as the diet "not working." These symptoms usually resolve within a week's time.

Personalize it. Start with the basics above *and*:

* If you're having trouble with autoimmune conditions, eliminate eggs, too.

* If you're prone to weight gain, eat less meat and heavier foods (ex: stews, chili), more vegetables and raw foods.

* If you're prone to weight loss or having trouble gaining weight, eat more meats and heavier foods (ex: stews, chili), less raw foods like salads.

* If you're generally healthy and wanting a boost in energy, try short-term fasts of 12–16 hours. Due to the circadian rhythm of the digestive tract, skipping dinner is best (as opposed to skipping breakfast). Try this 1–2 times a week. (This fast also means no supplements or beverages other than tea or water during the fasting time.)

Remember: One size doesn't fit all, even with whole foods diets. Consult with an integrative/functional medicine doctor, whole foods nutritionist, or health coach if you experience food reactions and/or have other special considerations. See **3. Give yourself permission to receive** for a list of resources.

How you eat is just as important as what you eat.

• Take a few deep, slow breaths before each meal. This stimulates the rest-and-digest nervous system.

• Chew your food. Whole foods require proper breakdown in order to release and absorb their goodness, and this starts with proper chewing.

• Appreciate the food before you, and the animals and plants that provide your nourishment. This connects us to life's cycles, something greater that we are all a part of.

• When you eat, just eat. Sit at the kitchen table. Make it a screen-free zone. No multitasking. A bonus: visualize your food and trace it from your mouth down to your stomach, breaking it down into steps (feel your teeth as you chew, your tongue lift up as you begin to swallow, your throat open up as the food moves to the back of your mouth, then feel your food travel down your esophagus). This helps reconnect the mind-body circuitry.

- When you're *almost* full, stop eating. To do this, you have to eat mindfully, or else you'll miss the subtle signals from your body.

Day 28...29...30. You've reached the finish line!

- Congratulate yourself and your coparticipants! Feeding your body with slow food is hard work.

- Slowly reintroduce foods. Ideally, one class at a time, in small portions, separated by three days (ex: when reintroducing soy, consider a meal seasoned with soy sauce versus eating a bowl of tofu).

- Monitor setbacks or flare-ups of old symptoms, and record them. If you have setbacks, eliminate that food or food group for the next few months, or until your health significantly improves. You can try reintroducing again at that time.

- Use the 30-day Reset Diet as a basis for your general eating. Like many integrative-functional medicine practitioners, I support the 80/20 rule. That is, for 80 percent of the time, stick to these guidelines. For the other 20 percent, perhaps when you're at social events or traveling or eating out, give yourself more freedom.

- Find your own balance and avoid dogma. Being too obsessive about food rules can counteract any healing you're aiming for. (See **7. Change your thoughts, change your genes** for strategies on how to break the unhealthy thought cycle.)

My favorite cookbooks and books on food:

- *The Longevity Kitchen* by Rebecca Katz (**http://www.rebecca katz.com**)

- *Practical Paleo* by Diane San Filippo (**http://www.balanced bites.com**)

- *Against All Grain* by Danielle Walker (**http://www.against allgrain.com**)

- *Food Rules* by Michael Pollan

- *What to Eat* by Marion Nestle

Other resources:

- **http://www.westonapricefoundation.org.** Newsletters, events, and podcasts on ancestral diets and lifestyles.

- **http://www.chriskresser.com.** A leading nutrition and health blog with well-researched information on whys and hows, as well as personalized diet plans.

- **http://www.threestonehearth.com.** A Bay Area kitchen cooperative for those looking for slow food for various therapeutic diets or general ancestral diets, as well as a community of like-minded folk.

10. Break old habits that no longer serve you.

Habits are often actions we do without thinking, what science terms "automaticity." They sound innocuous enough, until we realize we become what we repeatedly do. So let's make sure they serve our best interest. What served us well before may not serve us well now.

1. Write down some habits you know aren't supportive of your healing (ex: eating ice cream late at night, pulling all-nighters, smoking). Decide if any of those habits are changeable.

2. Don't force yourself to quit before you're ready, as resistance can make the habit stronger.

3. Find a new habit you enjoy, and replace the old one with this one.

4. Give the new habit 30 days. Set up a calendar and mark it off each day.

5. Find a buddy to keep you accountable, or to start the new habit with you.

6. Once you've completed the 30 days, evaluate whether you can do it for another 30.

7. Studies show it takes an average of 21 days to form a simple habit. Bigger changes require more time, 50 or 60 days, or even longer.

8. Don't beat yourself up if you give into your old habit. Simply and gently redirect yourself to the new healthier habit you've chosen.

11. Practice pleasure. It's serious work.

Play is my favorite prescription for patients. It can shift the mind and body from fight-or-flight to rest-and-digest, releasing endorphins (the body's natural painkillers), lowering blood pressure, and increasing immune function. Yet it is one of the most underrated activities in our work-driven culture, and when we feel threatened or stressed or unwell, play and pleasure are among the first things to go. If you're serious about healing, play needs to be a priority—even if at first it feels like work.

1. Make a list of things that once brought you pleasure. Choose 1 or 2 from that list and commit to doing them once a week, minimum (ex: reading books you once loved, caring for a pet, keeping fresh flowers in your room).

2. Go to YouTube and search under "funny videos." Watch a few and laugh along—whether your laughter is fake or genuine, it

doesn't matter. But you have to have a smile on your face and laugh from your belly for your body to release endorphins and other anti-inflammatory chemicals into your bloodstream.

3. Practice "laughter yoga" on your own.

    Clap your hands in a regular rhythm.

    Say "ho, ho, ha ha," in time to the clapping.

    Move around the room as you do this.

    Take deep breaths and release them with belly laughs.

    Do something playful—sing a cheerful song, dance naked to a song you love—and thank yourself for it when it's over.

12. Investigate hidden root causes.

A lot of the other How to Heal steps address root causes of chronic conditions: inadequate sleep, a sedentary lifestyle, poor nutrition or inadequate hydration, emotional and spiritual stress, social isolation, and pollutants. So, here, I'll focus on two big ones that are often overlooked: (1) food allergens, and (2) stealth infections.

Food Allergens

An allergy and a sensitivity are two different immune responses to foods. The testing for allergies is more reliable, with either blood or skin testing. You should eliminate the foods you are allergic to.

The testing of sensitivities, however, is notoriously fickle. Different practitioners recommend different ways to test sensitivities, but in the end, the best way is for you to do a trial elimination of the common culprits, then reintroduce them later, one by one, and see how you feel. See **9. Heal the gut** for more details. Gluten and dairy sensitivities don't always necessitate lifelong elimination; sometimes it just takes eliminating them long enough for your gut to heal and your immune system to quiet down, and then follow the 80/20 rule.

If you've tried the 30-Day Reset Diet, or another elimination diet, and are confused as to what to eat, or are having trouble reintroducing foods, seek out a dietary practitioner, many of whom work virtually. See **3. Give yourself permission to receive** for resources.

If you've tested positive for multiple allergies or sensitivities, this underscores the need for more comprehensive gut-healing and immune support.

Stealth Infections

These are viruses, bacteria, parasites, or yeasts that stimulate enough inflammation to cause symptoms or contribute to chronic disease, but not enough to be picked up by standard screening labs, per se. If you suspect this may be an issue for you, here are a few suggestions:

1. If you have experienced prolonged fatigue, ask your doctor to consider screening you for Epstein-Barr virus (EBV) for "reactivation syndrome." This is different than acute mono or past infection. You need the regular panel plus the "EA" or early antigen.

2. If you only have access to general labs like Quest or LabCorp, ask your doctor to consider screening you for parasites or disease-causing bacteria in the gut. This is a three-sample test. On the third sample, do a "purge." Get Natural Calm, a powder of magnesium citrate, online or from your local pharmacy. The night before your sample, take increments up to 8–10 tsp total of the Natural Calm powder. This should induce a loose or watery bowel movement in the morning, which may increase the yield of the sample. Drink lots of coconut water and broth and water to keep from getting dehydrated.

3. I strongly recommend you work with a functional medicine practitioner or a naturopath to do more testing, including Lyme and other tick-borne infections, chronic viruses, as well as toxic mold exposure. Each of these is an intensive area of diagnostics and treatment, so it's best to check if your doctor is

well-trained to treat these conditions. **5. Detoxify yourself** and **9. Heal the gut** are foundational to healing chronic infections, so those are good starting places.

My favorite resources:

- *Why Do I Still Have Thyroid Symptoms? When My Lab Tests Are Normal: A Revolutionary Breakthrough in Understanding Hashimoto's Disease and Hypothyroidism*, by Datis Kharrazian, PhD

- *Hashimoto's Thyroiditis: Lifestyle Interventions for Finding and Treating the Root Cause*, by Izabella Wentz, PhD

- Stanford Medicine ME/CFS Initiative, **http://www.med .stanford.edu/chronicfatiguesyndrome**

- Bay Area Lyme Foundation, **http://www.bayarealyme.org**

- Surviving Mold, **http://www.survivingmold.com**

- Phoenix Helix podcasts, **http://www.phoenixhelix.com**

13. Survive love and loss.

Grief and loss touch everyone. No one is exempt. By bringing grief out of the shadows, you remember your humanity, cleanse your soul, and make room for more love in your life. Not grieving risks suppression, while grieving alone risks depression.

Here are two simple but powerful exercises I learned from Francis Weller, the grief therapist. The ritual of speaking to the earth is common among many cultures around the world.

1. Timed automatic writings, to help you remember what has been buried.

   Find a friend or a family member whom you trust, in person or on the phone. Find a private space where you won't be interrupted.

   Decide on the length of time for the writing exercise (suggested: 5, 8, or 10 minutes).

Set the ground rules: complete confidentiality of what is shared.

Choose a starter phrase, which will be the thread in the exercise. Some examples: I remember when…, My tears…, I wish someone would…, What I meant was…

Once the exercise begins, each person must write continuously. No stopping, no crossing out, no erasing, no rereading. If your mind is a blank, you can write exactly that: My mind is a blank, *repeatedly, or* Nothing is coming up, Nothing is coming up… *until something comes up. By removing the capacity to edit yourself, you silence your judging mind and allow your soul or subconscious to emerge.*

When the designated amount of time is up, stop. Don't finish your sentence, or even cross your T. Sometimes you can glean significance from the precise point at which you stopped.

Take turns reading your words to each other. The listener practices "generous listening," which means full attention without interruptions, questions, or comments (if you find yourself forming a response in your mind, try to let those thoughts go; even approval is a form of judgment, because it shapes the other person's thoughts). When the reader is finished, the listener simply says "Thank you for sharing." Then switch roles.

You can end your session now, or repeat the exercise with a different starter phrase.

After you're finished, make an agreement: no sharing of what was read, and no referencing in the future, unless the reader himself or herself brings it up.

2. Speaking to the earth, to help you release grief from your body. You may do this alone, or invite witnesses to join you.

    Find a space in nature that feels completely safe: your sanctuary. It can be your backyard, a spot in a park, or a place in the wild. If you have ready access to a forest or a creek or a beach, feel those spaces out.

Dig a small opening in the earth or sand, large enough to speak into.

Feel the earth below you, allowing it to support all your weight.

Say your grief into the earth. Here is an example that Francis gives in his book, The Wild Edge of Sorrow: *"I have been carrying this grief for so long, and I cannot hold it any longer. It is too big for me. It is weighing me down and depriving me of any joy. I know you can hold this sorrow. In fact, you can turn it into something sweet for the roots that rest in your body. I do this to set down my sorrows so I can better participate in the mending of our community. Thank you for being here for me and all of us."*

If you're called to, lie down to speak or cry or scream your grief into the earth.

When you're done, fill the hole back up, returning it to its former shape, and thank the earth for being your holder.

My favorite books on grief and grieving:

- *The Wild Edge of Sorrow* by Francis Weller

- *Wild Mind: A Field Guide to the Human Psyche* by Bill Plotkin

- *Dark Nights of the Soul: A Guide to Finding Your Way Through Life's Ordeals* by Thomas Moore

14. Reclaim your purpose.

A sense of purpose can lead to a higher quality of life. But a chronic illness may challenge you to let go of what used to define you.

Look at what you love now. Start small, with what's in front of you: providing for your children, or contributing to small projects at home, or taking care of a pet.

If you have trouble, try **6. Let intuition tell your thinking mind where to look next**, or **7. Change your thoughts, change your genes**.

Sometimes what we need isn't more advice or more thoughts, but silence.

15. Find your story, the real one.

One of my mentors, Rachel Remen, MD, said that sometimes we may need a story more than food to live. Food and stories nourish us in different ways. A story allows us to give meaning to or explore in metaphor an experience that feels overwhelming, chaotic, or fragmented.

Here are some ideas to get you started, taken from writing assignments for Columbia University's Narrative Medicine program:

1. Come up with an idea for a short story of illness you want to tell.

2. Try writing the narrative in different forms—prose, poetry, or a play.

3. Try writing about the familial, cultural, or ethnic context of the illness story.

4. Write about how your body may be perceived by others, like your doctor.

5. Address the issue of bodily integration into self.

6. Give your story to a reader. For safety and support, it may be best to find a partner for this assignment, and to commit to confidentiality, no critiques, and no questions. As with the grieving process, a generous listener is the most healing reader.

Here are some general writing prompts, adapted from the Integrative Medicine Program at the University of Wisconsin-Madison School of Medicine and Public Health. These writing exercises are intended to be 5–10 minutes long.

1. Write about the origin of your name.

2. Write about one of your scars.

3. Write about the time someone took care of you.

4. Write about the time you took care of someone else.

My favorite resources for narrative writing:

- *The Art of Memoir* by Mary Karr

- *Telling True Stories*, edited by Mark Kramer and Wendy Call

- *The Illness Narratives: Suffering, Healing, and the Human Condition* by Arthur Kleinman

Additional Resources

1. Open Medicine Foundation, whose mission is to fund collaborative research of chronic complex diseases. See their "The End of ME/CFS Project" for more information. **www.omf.ngo**

2. Phoenix Rising, a nonprofit organization that provides information and new research to support health and well-being, and maintains one of the largest chronic fatigue syndrome forums in the world. **www.phoenixrising.me**

3. *Unrest*, a documentary film by Jennifer Brea that tells the backstory of patients with chronic fatigue syndrome, and calls for increased awareness and research.

4. Healing Circles, a global learning community committed to sharing resources for joining or facilitating support groups, centered on the whole person—mind, body, and spirit—and creating safe havens for exploration. **www.healingcircles global.org**

Gratitude

Because we don't heal alone.

—*Carl Jung*

Thank you, first and foremost, to my parents, Timothy and Ann Li, for traveling to the other side of the world to support me; for reading my first draft with courage; for making sacrifices that I could never know. To my sister, Sharon Leong, and my brother-in-law, Mark Leong, for your love while far and near; for your sharp minds and big hearts on this book; for helping me remember how things were. To my brothers, Patrick and David Li, and their wives, Camille and Alice Li, for your steadfastness and good humor. And to my niece and nephews— Edie, Oscar, Boris, and Edison—for filling our lives with joy.

To Adam and Arlie Hochschild—better parents, I couldn't have designed. Your close presence in our lives was a light in the darkness, and provided for Rosa and Sonia not only a sense of stability, but one of abundance; you were also indispensable teachers for how to tell a good story. To Gabriel Hochschild, my soul brother, for keeping me grounded with your pragmatic wisdom.

To friends who were invaluable readers: Salahuddin Kazi, Sanda Balaban, Meena Palaniappan, Jason Hanasik, Kat Toups, Ted Schettler, Deirdre English, Christina Desser, and Vindi Singh. To Bill Kelly, Zahra Ghayour-Kelly, David Tjen, Lynna Tsou, Sean Boyle, Ben and BeckiLynn Morgenthau, Irene Lee, Catharine Meyers, Elisabeth Ross, Christine Wang, Sandra Tsai, Devra Nelson, Lhakpa Dolma, Chao Wo Yip, Danae Husary, Lydia Gilbert, Sophia Weltman, Wayne Standerwick, Cassia Holstein, Olivia Rodberg for nourishing my family and me with your affection, prayers, home-cooked meals, Thai takeout, carpools, play, laughter, tears. To Juan Carlos Collins and Stefania Cargnello, whose abiding friendship shows me what "embodied souls" look like in their fullest.

To Judy and the late Robert Wey, for being my spiritual parents; for enduring life's challenges with such grace and resilience. I'm so glad Bob got to read the fuller account of Kurt, in all its glory and complexity. And to the memory of Kurt.

To my uncle Joseph Lee and my cousin Debbie Loh for your oral histories of my ancestors.

To Steve Heilig and the San Francisco Medical Society for publishing my personal essay, which was the seed for this book. To the "How to Write a Book" class at UC Berkeley's Graduate School of Journalism, taught by Adam Hochschild, for helping me mold the initial outlines of my book, before I knew what a narrative arc was and after my first elevator pitch broke me into sobs.

To the extraordinary team at New Harbinger, starting with Catharine Meyers and Matthew McKay, whose bold vision inspired this book. To my editors, Vicraj Gill, Georgia Kolias, and Teja Watson, who worked, then reworked every page with brilliance. I felt the entire team rooting not just for this project, but for me. I never imagined the publishing process could be so intimate, so gratifying.

To the Finding Meaning in Medicine circle, facilitated by Rachel Remen, for listening generously. To the Mysteria Circle—Alexandra Johnson, Rupa Marya, Deborah Cohan—for being my fellow doctor-mother-activist-intuitive sojourners; and for never telling. You humble and inspire me.

To my mentors—doctors, priests, health-care practitioners, therapists, many of whom I met after the time frame in this book—for paving the way as model healers. Rachel Remen, Yeshi Neumann, Martine Bloquiaux, Robert Levine, Carmen Hering, the late Pia Aitken, the late Seymour Eisenberg, the late Daniel Foster, Salahuddin Kazi, Francis Weller, Ted Schettler, Annie Hopper, Sunjya Schweig, Jennifer Poehler, Mona Moy, Mingtong Gu, Phil Brochard, Liz Tichenor. And to Paul Farmer, for being the kind of doctor I want to be when I finally grow up.

To Richard Rohr, whom I have never met, but whose daily meditations bring stunning clarity to my life.

To the Bay Area Functional Medicine group, facilitated by Kat Toups and Myrto Ashe, for keeping me ever learning. And to the pioneers at the Institute for Functional Medicine, especially Mark Hyman, Jeffrey Bland, David Jones, Datis Kharrazian, Robert Rountree, Patrick Hanaway, Mimi Guarneri, Michael Stone.

To Salahuddin (Dino) Kazi: the changes you've made to the internal medicine residency program at UT Southwestern are brilliant and important. Your friendship has been a continuous light in my life, and I look forward to the day when we share another glass of Ojai Syrah while listening to the Buena Vista Social Club and discussing a unified theory of knowledge.

To Charles Ho, for daring to love me as my eighteen-year-old self, big hair, big ego, and all. Your impromptu visit in 2017 was literally lifesaving. It brings me great solace and joy to know you're in my life.

To Michael Lerner, for reading draft upon draft of my book, for mentoring me in environmental health and integrative medicine, for exemplifying a life of service, but mostly, for the example of your being. Our walks and conversations are among my most beloved treasures.

Lastly, thank you to my husband, David Hochschild, and to our daughters, Rosa and Sonia. You guide me. You enliven me. There are no words, really. But in my mind's eye, I hold an image: a dolphin, a flying squirrel, and a rainbow bird, dancing about a hummingbird come back to life.

References

American Psychological Association. (2003). Marriage appears to be beneficial to women's health, but only when marital satisfaction is high, new research shows. Retrieved from http://www.apa.org/releases/maritalbenefit.html.

Basseri R. J., Weitsman, S., Barlow, G. M., & Pimentel, M. (2011). Antibiotics for the treatment of irritable bowel syndrome. *Gastroenterology and Hepatology, 7*, 455–493.

Bell, D. S., & Bell, D. E. (2010). Definition of recovery in chronic fatigue syndrome. *Journal of IiMe, 4*, 23–27.

Boyce, W. T., & Ellis, B. J. (2005). Biological sensitivity to context: Empirical explorations of an evolutionary-developmental theory. *Developmental Psychopathology, 17*, 303–328.

Bratic A., & Larsson, N. (2013). The role of mitochondria in aging. *Journal of Clinical Investigation, 123*, 951–957.

Burek C. L., & Talor, M. V. (2009). Environmental triggers of autoimmune thyroiditis. *Journal of Autoimmunity, 33*, 183–189.

Cairns R., & Hotopf, M. (2005). A systematic review describing the prognosis of chronic fatigue syndrome. *Occupational Medicine, 55*, 20–31.

Cao H., Pan, X., Hua, L., & Liu, J. (2009). Acupuncture for treatment of insomnia. *Journal of Alternative and Complementary Medicine, 15*, 1171–1186.

Carding, S., Verbeke, K., Vipond, D. T., Corfe, B. M., & Owen, L. J. (2015). Dysbiosis of the gut microbiota in disease. *Microbial Ecology in Health and Disease, 26*.

Ch'ng C. L., Jones, M. K., & Kingham, J. G. C. (2007). Celiac disease and autoimmune thyroid disease. *Clinical Medicine Research, 5*, 184–192.

Cotran R., Kumar, V., & Robbins, S. L. (1994). *Pathologic basis of disease* (5th ed.). Philadelphia, PA: W. B. Saunders Company.

Curley, J. P., Mashoodh, R., & Champagne, F. A. (2011). Epigenetics and the origins of paternal effects. *Hormones and Behavior, 59*, 306–314.

Dantzer, R., O'Connor, J. C., Freund, G. G., Johnson, R. W., & Kelley, K. W. (2008). From inflammation to sickness and depression: When the immune system subjugates the brain. *Nature Reviews Neuroscience, 9*, 46–56.

Devine, A. S., Jackson, C. S., Lyons, L., & Mason, J. D. (2010). Frequency of incidental findings on computed tomography of trauma patients. *Western Journal of Emergency Medicine, 11*, 24–27.

Doidge, N. (2007). *The brain that changes itself: Stories of personal triumph from the frontiers of brain science.* New York: Penguin Books.

Dube, S. R., Fairweather, D., Pearson, W. S., Felitti, V. J. Anda, R. F., & Croft, J. B. (2009). Cumulative childhood stress and autoimmune diseases in adults. *Psychosomatic Medicine, 71*, 243–250.

Eckle, T. (2015). Health impact and management of a disrupted circadian rhythm and sleep in critical illnesses. *Current Pharmaceutical Design, 21*, 3428–3430.

Enig, M. (2011). *Know your fats: The complete primer for understanding the nutrition of fats, oils, and cholesterol*. Silver Spring, MD: Bethesda Press.

Franke, H. A. (2014). Toxic stress: Effects, prevention, and treatment. *Children, 1*, 390–402.

Fredrick, J. F. (1977). Grief as a disease process. *Omega Journal of Death and Dying, 7*, 297–305.

Freeman, R., & Komaroff, A. L. (1997). Does the chronic fatigue syndrome involve the autonomic nervous system? *American Journal of Medicine, 102*, 357–364.

Fukuda, K., Straus, S. E., Hickie, I., Sharpe, M. C., Dobbins, J. G., & Komaroff, A. (1994). The chronic fatigue syndrome: A comprehensive approach to its definition and study. *Annals of Internal Medicine, 121*, 953–959.

Fujii, N., Tabira, T., Shibasaki, H., Kuroiwa, Y., Ohnishi, A., & Nagaki, J. (1982). Acute autonomic and sensory neuropathy associated with elevated Epstein-Barr virus antibody titre. *Journal of Neurology, Neuro- surgery, and Psychiatry, 45*, 656–658.

Gilhooly, P. E., Ottenweller, J. E., Lange, G., Tiersky, L., & Natelson, B. H. (2001). Chronic fatigue and sexual dysfunction in female Gulf War veterans. *Journal of Sex and Marital Therapy, 27*, 483–487.

Gladwell, V. F., Brown, D. K., Barton, J. L., Tarvainen, M. P., Kuoppa, P., Pretty, J., Suddaby, J. M., & Sandercock, G. R. (2012). The effects of views of nature on autonomic control. *European Journal of Applied Physiology, 112*, 3379–3386.

Hadjivassilou, M., Rao, D. G., Grinewald, R. A., Aeschlimann, D. P., Sarrigiannis, P. G., Hoggard, N. … Sanders, D. S. (2016). Neurological dysfunction in coeliac disease and non-coeliac gluten sensitivity. *American Journal of Gastroenterology, 111*, 561–567.

HeartMath Institute. (2010). New study further supports intuition. Retrieved from https://www.heartmath.org/articles-of-the-heart/science-of-the-heart/new-study -further-supports-intuition/.

Heim, C., Nater, U. M., Maloney, E., Boneva, R., Jones, J. F., & Reeves, W. C. (2009). Childhood trauma and risk for chronic fatigue syndrome. *Archives of General Psychiatry, 66*, 72–80.

Hoffmann, D. E., & Tarzian, A. J. (2001). The girl who cried pain: A bias against women in the treatment of pain. *Journal of Law, Medicine, and Ethics, 29*, 13–27.

Holt-Lundstad, J., Birmingham, W., & Jones, B. Q. (2008). Is there something unique about marriage? The relative impact of marital status, relationship quality, and network social support on ambulatory blood pressure and mental health. *Annals of Behavioral Medicine, 35*, 239–44.

Holt-Lunstad, J., Smith, T. B., & Layton, J. B. (2010). Social relationships and mortality risk: A meta-analytic review. *PLOS Med, 7*.

Hu, Y., Costenbader, K. H., Gao, X., Al-Daabil, M., Sparks, J. A., Solomon, D. H., … Lu, B. (2014). Sugar-sweetened soda consumption and risk of developing rheumatoid arthritis in women. *American Journal of Clinical Nutrition, 100*, 959–967.

Ingelfinger, F. J. (1980). Arrogance. *New England Journal of Medicine, 25*, 1507–1511.

Jackson, J. R., Eaton, W. W., Cascella, N. G., Fasano, A., & Kelly, D. L. (2012). Neurologic and psychiatric manifestations of celiac disease and gluten sensitivity. *Psychiatric Quarterly, 83*, 91–102.

Janegova, A., Janega, P., Rychly, B., Kuracinova, K., & Babal, P. (2015). The role of Epstein-Barr virus infection in the development of autoimmune thyroid diseases. *Endokrynologia Polska, 66*, 132–136.

Jessen, N. A., Munk, A. S., Lundgaard, I., & Nedergaard, M. (2015). The glymphatic system: A beginner's guide. *Neurochemical Research, 40*, 2583–2599.

Johnson, M. L., Robinson, M. M., & Nair, K. S. (2013). Skeletal muscle aging and the mitochondrion. *Trends in Endocrinology and Metabolism, 24*, 247–256.

Jones, D., Bland, J., & Quinn, S. (2010). What is functional medicine? In D. S. Jones & S. Quinn (Eds.,), *Textbook of functional medicine* (5–14). Gig Harbor, WA: The Institute for Functional Medicine.

Kajeepeta S., Gelaye, B., Jackson, C. L., & Williams, M. A. (2015). Adverse childhood experiences are associated with adult sleep disorders: A systematic review. *Sleep Medicine, 16*, 320–330.

Keely, E., J. (2011). Postpartum thyroiditis: An autoimmune thyroid disorder which predicts future thyroid health. *Obstetrics Medicine, 4*, 7–11.

Kellermann, N. P. (2013). Epigenetic transmission of Holocaust trauma: Can nightmares be inherited? *Israel Journal of Psychiatry and Related Sciences, 50*, 33–39.

Kharrazian, D. (2013). *Why isn't my brain working?: A revolutionary understanding of brain decline and effective strategies to recover your brain's health.* Carlsbad, CA: Elephant Press.

Kim, J. E., Seo, B. K, Choi, J. B., Kim, J. H., Kim, T. H, Lee, M. H. … Choi, S. M. (2015). Acupuncture for chronic fatigue syndrome and idiopathic chronic fatigue: A multicenter, nonblinded, randomized controlled trial. *Trials, 16*, 314.

Kim, T., Jeong, G. W., Baek, H. S., Kim, G. W., Sundaram, T., Kang, H. K., … Song, J. K. (2010). Human brain activation in response to visual stimulation with rural and urban scenery pictures: A functional magnetic resonance imaging study. *Science of the Total Environment, 408*, 2600–2607.

Kohlstadt, I. (Ed.). (2012). *Advancing Medicine with Food and Nutrients* (2nd ed.). Boca Raton, FL: CRC Press.

Koulivand, P. H., Ghadiri, M. K., & Gorji, A. (2013). Lavender and the nervous system. *Evidence-Based Complementary and Alternative Medicine, 2013.*

Kumar, S. (2016). Burnout and doctors: Prevalence, prevention, and intervention. *Healthcare, 4.*

Lieberman, D. (2014). *The story of the human body: Evolution, health, and disease.* New York: Vintage Books.

Ma., T., Liaset, B., Hao, Q., Petersen, R. K., Fjære, E., Ngo, H. T., … Madsen, L. (2011). Sucrose counteracts the anti-inflammatory effect of fish oil in adipose tissue and increases obesity development in mice. *PLoS One, 6.*

Mancini, A., Di Segni, C., Raimondo, S., Olivieri, G., Silvestrini, A., Meucci, E., & Currò, D. (2016). Thyroid hormones, oxidative stress, and inflammation. *Mediators of Inflammation, 2016.*

McDade, T. W., Rutherford, J., Adair, L., & Kuzawa, C. W. (2009). Early origins of inflammation: Microbial exposures in infancy predict lower levels of C-reactive protein in adulthood. *Proceedings of the Royal Society, 277,* 1129–1137.

Montoya, J. G., Kogelnik, A. M., Bhangoo, M., Lunn, M. R., Flamand, L., Merrihew, L. E., ... Desai, M. (2013). Randomized clinical trial to evaluate the efficacy and safety of valganciclovir in a subset of patients with chronic fatigue syndrome. *Journal of Medical Virology, 85,* 2101–2109.

Moslehi, N. Mohammadreza, V., Rahimi-Fouroushani, A., & Banafsheh, G. (2012). Effects of oral magnesium supplementation on inflammatory markers in middle-aged overweight women. *Journal of Research in Medical Sciences, 17,* 607–614.

Mullington, J. M., Simpson, N. S., Meier-Ewert, H. K., & Haack, M. (2010). Sleep loss and inflammation. *Best Practice and Research: Clinical Endocrinology and Metabolism, 24,* 775–784.

Nakatomi, Y., Mizuno, K., Ishii, A., Wada, Y., Tanaka, M., Tazawa, S., ... Watanabe, Y. (2014). Neuroinflammation in patients with chronic fatigue syndrome/myalgic encephalomyelitis. *Journal of Nuclear Medicine, 55,* 945–950.

National Institute for Health and Care Excellence. (2007). Chronic fatigue syndrome/ myalgic encephalomyelitis (or encephalopathy): diagnosis and management of chronic fatigue syndrome/myalgic encephalomyelitis (or encephalopathy) in adults and children. Retrieved from https://www.nice.org.uk/guidance/cg53 /evidence/full-guideline-pdf-196524109.

Naschitz, J. E., Yeshurun, D., & Rosner, I. (2004). Dysautonomia in chronic fatigue syndrome: Facts, hypotheses, implications. *Medical Hypotheses, 62,* 203–206.

Newman, T. (2016). *Inflammation turns mitochondria into toxic factories.* Retrieved from http://www.medicalnewstoday.com/articles/313090.php.

O'Connor, M. F., Irwin, M. R., & Wellisch, D. K. (2009). When grief heats up: Pro-inflammatory cytokines predict regional brain activity. *Neuroimage, 47,* 891–896.

O'Rourke, M. (2014). Doctors tell all—and it's bad. *The Atlantic.* Retrieved from https://www.theatlantic.com/magazine/archive/2014/11/doctors-tell-all-and-its -bad/380785.

Orloff, J. (2010). *Second sight: An intuitive psychiatrist tells her extraordinary story and shows you how to tap your own inner wisdom.* New York: Three Rivers Press.

Palma, B. D., Gabriel, A., Colugnati, F. A., & Tufik, S. (2006). Effects of sleep deprivation on the development of autoimmune disease in an experimental model of systemic lupus erythematosus. *American Journal of Physiology: Regulatory, Integrative, and Comparative Physiology, 291,* R1527–R1532.

Papadopoulos, A. S. , & Cleare, A. J. (2011). Hypothalamic–pituitary–adrenal axis dysfunction in chronic fatigue syndrome. *Nature Review Endocrinology, 27,* 22–32.

Park, S. H., & Mattson, R. H. (2009). Ornamental indoor plants in hospital rooms enhanced health outcomes of patients recovering from surgery. *Journal of Alternative and Complementary Medicine, 15,* 975–980.

Pearce, E. N., & Braverman, L. E. (2009). Environmental pollutants and the thyroid. *Best Practices and Research: Clinical Endocrinology and Metabolism, 23,* 801–813.

Pongratz, G., & Straub, R. H. (2014). The sympathetic nervous response in inflammation. *Arthritis Research and Therapy, 16.*

Potera C. (2010). Diet and nutrition: The artificial food dye blues. *Environmental Health Perspectives, 118.*

Price, W. A. (2009). *Nutrition and physical degeneration.* Lemon Grove, CA: Price Pottenger Nutrition Foundation.

Rao, A. V., Bested, A. C., Beaulne, T. M., Katzman, M. A., Iorio, C., Berardi, J. M., & Logan, A. C. (2009). A randomized, double-blind, placebo-controlled pilot study of a probiotic in emotional symptoms of chronic fatigue syndrome. *Gut Pathogens, 1.*

Rodríguez, J. M., Murphy, K., Stanton, C., Ross, R. P., Kober, O. I., Juge, N., ... Collado, M. C. (2015). The composition of the gut microbiota throughout life, with an emphasis on early life. *Microbial Ecology in Health and Disease, 26.*

Rosanoff, A., Weaver, C. M., & Rude, R. K. (2012). Suboptimal magnesium status in the United States: Are the health consequences underestimated? *Nutrition Reviews, 70,* 153–164.

Salim, S., Chugh, G., & Asghar, M. (2012). Inflammation in anxiety. *Advances in Protein Chemistry and Structural Biology, 88,* 1–25.

Schultze-Florey, C. R., Martinez-Maza, O., Magpantay, L., Breen, E. C., Irwin, M. R., Gündel, H., & O'Connor, M. F. 2012. When grief makes you sick: Bereavement-induced systemic inflammation is a question of genotype. *Brain, Behavior, and Immunity, 26,* 1066–1071.

Shanafelt, T. D., Boone, S., Tan, L., Dyrbye, L. N., Sotile, W., Satele, D., ... Oreskovich, M. R. (2012). Burnout and satisfaction with work-life balance among US physicians relative to the general US population. *Archives of Internal Medicine, 172,* 1377–1385.

Srivastava J. K., Shankar, E., & Gupta, S. (2010). Chamomile: An herbal medicine of the past with a bright future. *Molecular Medicine Reports, 3,* 895–901.

Stagnaro-Green, A. (2004). Postpartum thyroiditis. *Best Practice and Research: Clinical Endocrinology and Metabolism, 18,* 303–316.

Steenland, K., Fletcher, T., & Savitz, D. A. (2010). Epidemiologic evidence on the health effects of perfluorooctanoic acid (PFOA). *Environmental Health Perspectives, 118,* 1100–1108.

Stojanovich, L., & Marisavljevich, D. (2008). Stress as a trigger of autoimmune disease. *Autoimmunity Reviews, 7,* 209–213.

The future of healthcare: A national survey of physicians. Accessed 12 Dec 2018. Retrieved from http://www.thedoctors.com/about-the-doctors-company/news room/the-future-of-healthcare-survey/

The surprising dangers of CT scans and x-rays. *Consumer Reports.* Published 27 Jan 2015. Retrieved from http://www.consumerreports.org/cro/magazine/2015/01/the -surprising-dangers-of-ct-sans-and-x-rays/index.htm.

Thorley-Lawson, D. A., Babcock, G. J. (1999). A model for persistent infection with Epstein-Barr virus: The stealth virus of human B cells. *Life Sciences, 65,* 1433–1453.

Thyroid disease: understanding hypothyroidism and hyperthyroidism. Published 5 Aug 2015. *Harvard Health Publishing website.*

University of California Riverside. Published 17 Aug 2017. Three factors could explain physician burnout in the US. http://www.sciencedaily.com/releases/2018/08/180817125341.htm.

Van Heukelom, R. O., Prins, J. B., Smits, M. G., & Bleijenberg, G. (2006). Influence of melatonin on fatigue severity in patients with chronic fatigue syndrome and late melatonin secretion. *European Journal of Neurology, 13*, 55–60.

Virgin, H. W., Wherry, J., & Ahmed, R. (2009). Redefining chronic viral infection. *Cell, 138*, 30–50.

Weller, F. (2015). *The wild edge of sorrow: Rituals of renewal and the sacred work of grief.* Berkeley, CA: North Atlantic Books.

Wentz, I. (2013). *Hashimoto's thyroiditis: Lifestyle interventions for finding and treating the root cause.* Niwot, CO: Wentz, LLC.

Weyand, C. M., & Goronzy, J. J. (1992). Clinically silent infections in patients with oligoarthritis: Results of a prospective study. *Annals of the Rheumatic Diseases, 51*, 253–258.

WHO European Centre for Environment and Health. (2011). Burden of disease from environmental noise. Retrieved from http://www.euro.who.int/__data/assets/pdf_file/0008/136466/e94888.pdf.

Williams, F. (2005, January 9). Toxic breast milk? *New York Times Magazine.* Retrieved from http://www.nytimes.com/2005/01/09/magazine/toxic-breast-milk.html.

Yehuda R., & Lerner, A. (2018). Intergenerational transmission of trauma effects. *World Psychiatry, 17*, 243–257.

Youssef, N. A., Lockwood, L., Su, S., Hao, G., & Rutten, B. P. F. (2018). The effects of trauma, with or without PTSD, on the transgenerational DNA methylation alterations in human offsprings. *Brain Science, 8.*

Yuan, J., Gao, J., Li, X., Liu, F., Wijmenga, C., Chen, H., & Gilissen, L. J. W. J. (2013). The tip of the "celiac iceberg" in China. *PLoS One, 8.*

Zaletel, K., & Gaberšček, S. (2011). Hashimoto's thyroiditis: From genes to the disease. *Current Genomics, 12*, 576–588.

Cynthia Li, MD, graduated from the University of Texas Southwestern Medical Center, and has practiced internal medicine in settings as diverse as Kaiser Permanente Medical Center, San Francisco General Hospital, and St. Anthony Medical Clinic for the homeless. She currently serves on the faculty of the Healer's Art program at the UCSF School of Medicine, and has a private practice in integrative and functional medicine. She lives in Berkeley, CA, with her husband and their two daughters.

Foreword writer Arlie Russell Hochschild, PhD, is a sociologist and author of *Strangers in Their Own Land*.

MORE BOOKS

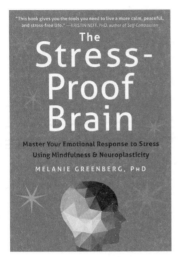

ISBN: 978-1626252660 | US $17.95

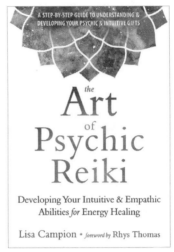

ISBN: 978-1684031214 | US $19.95

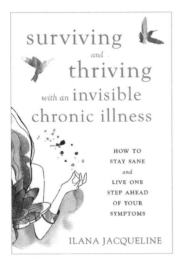

ISBN: 978-1626255999 | US $16.95

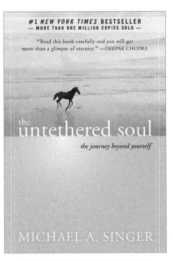

ISBN: 978-1572245372 | US $17.95

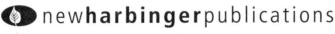